Fundamentals of Airway Surgery, Part I

Editors

JEAN DESLAURIERS

FARID M. SHAMJI

BILL NELEMS

THORACIC SURGERY CLINICS

www.thoracic.theclinics.com

Consulting Editor

M. BLAIR MARSHALL

May 2018 • Volume 28 • Number 2

ELSEVIER

1600 John F. Kennedy Boulevard • Suite 1800 • Philadelphia, Pennsylvania, 19103-2899

http://www.thoracic.theclinics.com

THORACIC SURGERY CLINICS Volume 28, Number 2
May 2018 ISSN 1547-4127, ISBN-13: 978-0-323-58376-3

Editor: John Vassallo (j.vassallo@elsevier.com)
Developmental Editor: Laura Fisher

Thoracic Surgery Clinics (ISSN 1547-4127) is published quarterly by Elsevier Inc., 360 Park Avenue South, New York, NY 10010-1710. Months of publication are February, May, August, and November. Business and editorial offices: 1600 John F. Kennedy Boulevard, Suite 1800, Philadelphia, PA 19103-2899. Periodicals postage paid at New York, NY, and additional mailing offices. Subscription prices are $373.00 per year (US individuals), $558.00 per year (US institutions), $100.00 per year (US students), $455.00 per year (Canadian individuals), $721.00 per year (Canadian institutions), $225.00 per year (Canadian and international students), $470.00 per year (international individuals), and $721.00 per year (international institutions). Foreign air speed delivery is included in all Clinics' subscription prices. All prices are subject to change without notice. **POSTMASTER:** Send address changes to Thoracic Surgery Clinics, Elsevier Health Sciences Division, Subscription Customer Service, 3251 Riverport Lane, Maryland Heights, MO 63043. **Customer Service (orders, claims, online, change of address): Telephone: 1-800-654-2452 (U.S. and Canada); 314-447-8871 (outside U.S. and Canada). Fax: 314-447-8029. E-mail: journalscustomerservice-usa@elsevier.com (for print support); journalsonlinesupport-usa@elsevier.com (for online support).**

Reprints. For copies of 100 or more, of articles in this publication, please contact Commercial Rights Department, Elsevier Inc., 360 Park Avenue South, New York, NY 10010-1710. Tel: 212-633-3874; Fax: 212-633-3820; E-mail: reprints@elsevier.com.

Thoracic Surgery Clinics is covered in *MEDLINE/PubMed (Index Medicus), EMBASE/Excerpta Medica, Science Citation Index Expanded (SciSearch®), Journal Citation Reports/Science Edition,* and *Current Contents®/Clinical Medicine.*

Contributors

CONSULTING EDITOR

M. BLAIR MARSHALL, MD, FACS
Chief, Division of Thoracic Surgery, Associate
Professor, Department of Surgery,
Georgetown University Medical Center,
Georgetown University School of Medicine,
Washington, DC, USA

EDITORS

JEAN DESLAURIERS, MD, FRCS(C), CM
Professor Emeritus, Laval University,
Quebec City, Quebec, Canada

FARID M. SHAMJI, MBBS, FRCSC, FACS
Professor of Surgery, Division of Thoracic
Surgery, The Ottawa Hospital–General
Campus, Ottawa, Ontario, Canada

[†]**BILL NELEMS, MD, FRCSC, MEd**
Professor Emeritus, Department of Surgery,
University of British Columbia, Vancouver,
Canada

AUTHORS

BENOIT JACQUES BIBAS, MD
Attending Thoracic, Division of Thoracic
Surgery, Heart Institute Hospital das Clinicas
da Faculdade de Medicina da Universidade de
Sao Paulo (InCor-HCFMUSP), Sao Paulo,
Sao Paulo, Brazil

**PAULO FRANCISCO GUERREIRO CARDOSO,
MD, MSc, PhD**
Attending Thoracic Surgeon, Collaborating
Professor, Division of Thoracic Surgery, Heart
Institute Hospital das Clinicas da Faculdade de
Medicina da Universidade de Sao Paulo
(InCor-HCFMUSP), Sao Paulo, Sao Paulo,
Brazil

JOEL D. COOPER, MD
Professor of Surgery, Hospital of the University
of Pennsylvania, University of Pennsylvania,
Philadelphia, Pennsylvania, USA

JEAN DESLAURIERS, MD, FRCS(C), CM
Professor Emeritus, Laval University,
Quebec City, Quebec, Canada

LAURA DONAHOE, MD
Division of Thoracic Surgery, Toronto General
Hospital, Toronto, Ontario, Canada

RICHARD J. FINLEY, MD, FRCSC, FACS
Emeritus Professor of Surgery, University of
British Columbia, Vancouver, British Columbia,
Canada

**PATRICK GULLANE, CM, OONT, MD,
FRCSC, FACS, FRACS(Hon), FRCS(Hon),
FRCSI(Hon)**
Wharton Chair in Head and Neck Surgery,
Department of Otolaryngology–Head and Neck
Surgery, University Health Network, University
of Toronto, Toronto, Ontario, Canada

[†]Deceased

WAEL HASAN, MB,BCh, LRCP & SI, BAO, NUI, MCh, MRCSI
Clinical Fellow in Head and Neck Oncology Surgery, Department of Otolaryngology–Head and Neck Surgery, University Health Network, University of Toronto, Toronto, Ontario, Canada

SHAF KESHAVJEE, MD
Division of Thoracic Surgery, Toronto General Hospital, Toronto, Ontario, Canada

PARESH MANE, MD, MCh
Attending Thoracic Surgeon, St Peters Hospital, Albany, New York, USA

DOUGLAS MATHISEN, MD
Hermes C. Grillo Professor of Thoracic Surgery, Chief, General Thoracic Surgery, Massachusetts General Hospital, Harvard Medical School, Boston, Massachusetts, USA

DONNA E. MAZIAK, MDCM, MSc, FRCSC, FACS
Surgical Oncology, Division of Thoracic Surgery, Ottawa Hospital–General Division, Professor, University of Ottawa, Ottawa, Ontario, Canada

MICHEAL C. McINNIS, MD
Joint Department of Medical Imaging, University Health Network, Mount Sinai Hospital, Women's College Hospital, Department of Medical Imaging, University of Toronto, Toronto, Ontario, Canada

REZA J. MEHRAN, MDCM, MSc, FRCSC, FACS
Professor, Department of Thoracic Surgery, The University of Texas MD Anderson Cancer Center, Houston, Texas, USA

HELIO MINAMOTO, MD, PhD
Attending Thoracic Surgeon, Collaborating Professor, Division of Thoracic Surgery, Heart Institute Hospital das Clinicas da Faculdade de Medicina da Universidade de Sao Paulo (InCor-HCFMUSP), Sao Paulo, Sao Paulo, Brazil

PHILIPPE MONNIER, MD
Professor Emeritus, Otolaryngology–Head and Neck Surgery Department, University Hospital CHUV, Lausanne, Switzerland

DARROCH MOORES, MD, FRCSC, FACS
Clinical Associate Professor of Surgery, Albany Medical College, Albany, New York, USA

PAULO MANUEL PÊGO-FERNANDES, MD, PhD
Professor, Head, Division of Thoracic Surgery, Heart Institute Hospital das Clinicas da Faculdade de Medicina da Universidade de Sao Paulo (InCor-HCFMUSP), Sao Paulo, Sao Paulo, Brazil

RAJAN SANTOSHAM, MS, MCh, FRCS
Head, Department of Thoracic Surgery, Santosham Chest Hospital, Chennai, India

HEIDI SCHMIDT, MD
Professor of Radiology, Department of Medical Imaging, University of Toronto, Joint Department of Medical Imaging, University Health Network, Mount Sinai Hospital, Women's College Hospital, Toronto, Ontario, Canada

FARID M. SHAMJI, MBBS, FRCSC, FACS
Professor of Surgery, Division of Thoracic Surgery, The Ottawa Hospital–General Campus, Ottawa, Ontario, Canada

THOMAS R.J. TODD, MD, FRCSC
Physician Advisor, The Canadian Medical Protective Association, Ottawa, Canada

GORDON WEISBROD, MD
Professor of Radiology, Department of Medical Imaging, University of Toronto, Joint Department of Medical Imaging, University Health Network, Mount Sinai Hospital, Women's College Hospital, Toronto General Hospital, Toronto, Ontario, Canada

CAMERON D. WRIGHT, MD
Division of Thoracic Surgery, Massachusetts General Hospital, Mathisen Family Professor of Surgery, Harvard Medical School, Boston, Massachusetts, USA

Contents

General Considerations

> Significant developments in airway surgery occurred following the introduction of mechanical ventilators and intubation with cuffed endotracheal tubes during the poliomyelitis epidemic of the 1950s. The resulting plethora of postintubation injuries provided extensive experience with resection and reconstruction of stenotic tracheal lesions. In the early 1960s, it was thought that no more than 2 cm of trachea could be removed. By the late 1960s, this was challenged owing to better knowledge of airway anatomy and blood supply, tension-releasing maneuvers, and improved anesthetic techniques. Currently, about half of the tracheal length can be safely removed and continuity restored by primary anastomosis.

> The surgical anatomy of the airways from the glottis to segmental bronchi is reviewed with a focus on pertinent anatomic findings surrounding common surgical procedures. The knowledge of the anatomy of the trachea while performing tracheostomy, tracheal and sleeve carinal resection, and bronchoplastic procedures is addressed. Pertinent anatomic relationships as evident on common computed tomographic imagery are emphasized.

> Advanced imaging plays an increasingly important role in the evaluation of the trachea. The use of computed tomography (CT) has evolved to include multiplanar reconstructions and 3-dimensional reconstructions for the evaluation of benign and malignant disease of the trachea. Advanced applications of CT include dynamic expiratory imaging for the diagnosis of tracheomalacia and virtual endoscopy as a complementary or alternative examination to flexible bronchoscopy. MRI of the trachea has limited applications but may see increased use in the future.

Surgical Disorders of the Airway

> Respiratory care advances such as the introduction of ventilatory assistance have been associated with postintubation airway stenosis resulting from tracheal injury

at the site of the inflatable cuff on endotracheal or tracheostomy tubes. Low-pressure cuffs have significantly reduced this occurrence. Loss of airway stability at the site of a tracheostomy stoma may result in tracheal stenosis. Subglottic stenosis may result from a high tracheostomy site at, or just inferior to, the cricoid arch, or to malposition of an endotracheal tube cuff. Awareness of these complications and their causes is essential to prevent their occurrence.

Surgery of the Proximal Airway

Idiopathic laryngotracheal stenosis is a rare but well-described indication for subglottic tracheal resection. Initially described by Pearson in 1975, the 1-stage subglottic tracheal resection with reconstruction of the airway ensures preservation of the recurrent laryngeal nerves while resulting in an effective and durable repair of the stenosis.

The management of pediatric laryngotracheal stenosis remains a challenging problem for the surgeon. The complexity of the various preoperative situations implies that no single treatment modality can solve the problem. This article focuses on the yield of partial cricotracheal resection and extended cricotracheal resection for the most severe grades of stenosis. Overall decannulation rates of 95% and 100% can be expected for isolated subglottic stenosis in patients with and without comorbidities but only 68% and 90% for patients with glotto-subglottic stenosis, respectively. Predictors of less favorable outcomes are severity of the stenosis, glottic involvement, and presence of comorbidities.

Optimal management of tracheal stenosis depends on identifying causative factors. Risk factors include high tracheostomy, cricothyroidotomy, prolonged intubation, and proximal migration of an endotracheal tube cuff. Management ranges from conservative observation to endoscopic procedures or open surgical resections. The goal of surgical repair is an adequate airway, decannulation, and normal laryngeal function. For early-stage disease, management of refractory conditions is via endoscopic procedures. An understanding of the respiratory function of the glottis and subglottis is essential when an optimum functional reconstruction of the glottic and subglottic area is considered. In this article, the authors discuss different airway assessments and surgical management techniques.

Tracheal disease is an infrequent problem requiring surgery. A high index of suspicion is necessary to correctly diagnose the problems. Primary concerns are safe control and assessment of the airway, familiarity with the principles of airway surgery, preserving tracheal blood supply, and avoiding anastomotic tension. A precise reproducible anastomotic technique must be mastered. Operation requires close cooperation with a knowledgeable anesthesia team. The surgeon must understand how to achieve the least tension on the anastomosis to avoid. It is advisable to examine the airway before discharge to check for normal healing and airway patency.

The factors governing successful healing of and impairing of tracheal and bronchial anastomosis are best understood by reviewing the normal histologic changes accompanying healing, governing factors, and biochemical advances made in the last 5 decades. Normal wound healing factors, also relevant to tracheal and bronchial reconstruction, rely on precise handling of tissues without interfering with tissue perfusion, careful selection and placement of sutures, and steps to minimize tension. Impairments of satisfactory healing are well recognized in gastrointestinal surgery and apply to tracheal and carinal resection and sleeve bronchial resection.

The ability to remove longer segments of airway and to extend resections into the larynx proper has managed to create novel situations that require attention to postoperative management. This article deals with prophylactic measures to prevent the requirement of assisted ventilation. It, however, also emphasizes various bronchoscopic and intubation techniques that, if required, help one to avoid trauma to the airway anastomosis. In addition, a variety of ventilator modalities are discussed that were developed by the author over many years at the Toronto General Hospital.

Tracheal resections are major surgical procedures with a complication rate as high as 44%. Early detection of complications followed by a structured and expedited course of action is critical for achieving a successful outcome. The prevention of complications after tracheal resection starts with a correct indication for resection. A thorough preoperative evaluation, meticulous surgical technique, and good postoperative care in a center that performs airway surgery routinely are important factors for achieving good results.

Modern thoracic surgery requires knowledge and skill in advanced bronchoscopic techniques. Rigid bronchoscopy remains a workhorse for the management of central airway obstruction. Dilation of tracheal strictures is now much simpler with the advent of the balloon dilator, which can be passed through a therapeutic bronchoscope. Numerous adjuncts, such as laser, argon beam coagulation, electrocautery, and cryotherapy, can be used to improve airway patency. There are now numerous stenting options for strictures that require stenting to maintain airway patency.

THORACIC SURGERY CLINICS

THE CLINICS ARE AVAILABLE ONLINE!
Access your subscription at:
www.theclinics.com

THORACIC SURGERY CLINICS

RELATED INTEREST

Preface
Fundamentals of Airway Surgery, Part I

This two-part miniseries on the "Fundamentals of Airway Surgery" was specifically conceived to honor the memory of Dr Frederick Griffith (Griff) Pearson (**Figs. 1** and **2**), who passed away in his 90th year on August 3, 2016. Dr Pearson dedicated much of his professional life to the advancement of airway surgery, not only in his native country, Canada, but also worldwide.

As will be appreciated through the reading of the articles concerning Dr Pearson in this issue, he was a most important contributor not only to the birth of airway surgery but also to its evolution over the past 60 years. It was indeed Dr Pearson who, along with Dr Hermes C. Grillo from Boston, recognized that endotracheal or tracheostomy tubes with high cuff pressures were largely responsible for the plethora of tracheal injuries that occurred following the worldwide epidemic of poliomyelitis that occurred in the early 1950s and signaled the birth of airway surgery. These observations are dutifully recorded by his long-time friend, Dr Joel Cooper, in his article.

After having systematically studied the laryngotracheal junction anatomy, Dr Pearson also described the "Pearson Operation," a procedure that allowed for the preservation of the recurrent nerves during the resection of subglottic strictures. The "Pearson operation" is now acknowledged as one of the most significant contributions of all time to airway surgery. A detailed description of the procedure can be found in the articles by Drs Keshavjee and Donahoe, Dr Monnier, and Drs Hasan and Gullane. All of this pioneering work led directly to the creation and successes of the "Lung Transplant Program" at the University of Toronto.

From our perspective as airway surgeons, we have elected to discuss in this issue those fundamental aspects of airway surgery that are so important to its successes, such as anatomy of the tracheobronchial tree, advanced technologies currently available to image it, and importance not only of anesthesia but also of maintaining high levels of communication between anesthesiologists and surgeons during surgery (see the articles by Dr Mehran and Drs McInnis, Weisbrod, and

Schmidt). Over the years, controversy has persisted over the length of airway that can be safely circumferentially resected, and in 1960, for instance, it was generally accepted that airway surgeons could safely remove no more than two to three tracheal rings ("The 2-cm Rule") and predictably be able to successfully reconstruct the airway with primary anastomosis. By the late 1960s, this 2-cm rule was being challenged due to improved knowledge of airway anatomy and blood supply as well as more liberal use of "tension-releasing maneuvers." About half of the tracheal length can now be safely removed and continuity restored by primary anastomosis with a minimum of morbidity, as discussed in the articles by Dr Mathisen, Dr Shamji, Dr Todd, and Dr Cardoso and colleagues, and by Dr Wright's article on nonoperative endoscopic management of benign tracheobronchial disorders. In order to have a complete text on the "Fundamentals of Airway Surgery," we finally elected to include essays regarding some uncommon surgical airway disorders, such as neoplasms, granulomatous diseases, and expiratory collapse (in the articles by Dr Cooper, Dr Maziak, Drs Moores and Mane, and Drs Santosham and Deslauriers, and in Dr Wright's article on tracheobronchomalacia and expiratory collapse of central airways).

Dr Pearson had a profound influence on the lives and professional careers of all of the authors of this issue of *Thoracic Surgery Clinics*. Indeed, authors were selected not only because they have a special expertise in airway surgery but also because were either trained by Dr Pearson or were close friends of his. Interestingly, authors come from nearly every corner of the world.

While planning the miniseries, we wanted to hire the services of expert medical artists to redraw all sketches, thus insuring uniformity throughout both issues. At the suggestion of the wife (Debbie Deslauriers) of one of the editors, we however changed our minds and agreed that it might be better to allow each author to express her or his thinking and what she or he may have learned while studying with Dr Pearson through personally made sketches. We felt that this would be more representative of the

Thorac Surg Clin 28 (2018) xi–xii
https://doi.org/10.1016/j.thorsurg.2018.02.004
1547-4127/18/© 2018 Published by Elsevier Inc.

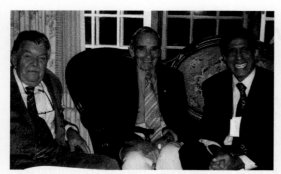

Fig. 1. From left to right: Drs Jean Deslauriers, F.G. Pearson, and Farid Shamji.

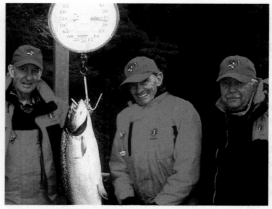

Fig. 2. From left to right: Drs Bill Nelems, F.G. Pearson, and Jean Deslauriers.

"Pearson Spirit." We also encouraged authors to quote, as much as possible, articles that had been written by Dr Pearson, and to this effect, we circulated to each one of them a complete list of Dr Pearson's publications.

In this preface, we also wish to honor the memory of Dr Bill Nelems (see **Fig. 2**), one of the coeditors of the miniseries, who passed away in March 2017 before he could complete the editing of the issues. Dr Nelems was a "master thoracic surgeon" who worked with Dr Pearson for several years and was very instrumental in helping him develop his expertise in airway surgery.

Obviously some real progress has been made in airway surgery since the beginning in the 1960s, but major challenges remain, including those of airway transplantation, use of airway prosthesis, and tracheal tissue regeneration, all issues that are discussed in part two of the miniseries.

In closing, we want to acknowledge that we are most grateful to Dr Blair Marshall, Consulting Editor for *Thoracic Surgery Clinics*, and John Vassallo, Associate Publisher at Elsevier, for their open minds on the idea of publishing a two-part miniseries on the "Fundamentals of Airway Sur-

gery" to honor Dr Pearson's memory. We would also like to thank and commend our Developmental Editors, Colleen Dietzler and Laura Fisher, whose acceptance of our inexperience with high technology and delays in production made our lives a lot easier over the past couple of years.

Jean Deslauriers, MD, FRCS(C), CM
Laval University
6364, Chemin Royal
Saint-Laurent-de-l'Île-d'Orléans
Quebec City, Quebec G0 A3Z0, Canada

Farid M. Shamji, MBBS, FRCSC
Division of Thoracic Surgery
The Ottawa Hospital–General Campus
501 Smyth Road
Ottawa, Ontario K1H 8L6, Canada

E-mail addresses:
jean.deslauriers@chg.ulaval.ca (J. Deslauriers)
fshamji@toh.ca (F.M. Shamji)

Dedication
Tribute to Frederick Griffith Pearson (1926–2016)

Dr Frederick Griffith Pearson (**Fig. 1**) was a remarkable surgeon, teacher, mentor, and leader. Griff was born and raised in Toronto as the son of an optometrist and an enlightened mother. A bright student, he attended the University of Toronto School, where his science teacher, Dr A.G. Kroll, encouraged him to become a physician. In 1949, he graduated as the silver medalist in Medicine at the University of Toronto. After his internship at the Toronto General Hospital (TGH), he spent a year in general practice in Port Colbourne. He then returned to the University of Toronto, where he did research under Wilfred G. Bigelow, studying hypothermia for cardiac surgery and the "mysteries of hibernation." His love of the Canadian North drew him to the secluded town of Wawa, Ontario for three years where the lack of speciality care exposed him to all aspects of Medicine, Surgery, and Obstetrics. He thrived in this environment and developed his great sense of always putting the patient first. In 1955, he returned to complete his General Surgery residency at the University of Toronto. In 1957, while a resident, he first became interested in tracheal stenosis secondary to tracheostomies, when he represented Surgery in the establishment of a four-bed respiratory failure unit at TGH, the first in Canada.

After becoming a Fellow of the Royal College of Physicians and Surgeons of Canada in 1958, he was advised by Drs Fred Kergin and Robert Janes to pursue further studies in tracheobronchial, pulmonary, and esophageal surgery. He received a McLaughlin traveling fellowship that allowed him to work with Mr Ronald Belsey at the Frenchay Hospital in Bristol. Not only did Mr Belsey teach Griff the nuances of esophageal surgery, he engrained in him the importance of careful lifelong follow-up of patients undergoing new operations. The information garnered from these clinics allowed Griff to improve on Mr Belsey's Mark IV hiatus hernia operation by adding the Collis gastroplasty to lengthen the esophagus of patients with a foreshortened esophagus.

In 1960, he travelled to Copenhagen to learn about prolonged mechanical ventilation by positive pressure ventilation. He observed severe injuries to the larynx and trachea that led him to develop a lifelong interest in tracheal and laryngeal surgery. At the main hospital in the Copenhagen, he met a young man named Astrup, who designed a technique to measure oxygen tension from a fingerprint in children. In those days, oxygen saturation was measured using the Van Slyke method that took hours, was very crude, and was not very accurate.

At the Karolinska Institute in Stockholm, he was sitting in the surgeons lounge between cases and met a pleasant young man who came in and spoke English very well. He introduced himself as Eric Carlens. Griff was familiar with the Carlens double-lumen endotracheal tube used for single-lung ventilation during thoracotomies. Griff asked, "Are you by chance related to the Carlens of the Carlens tube?" He looked at Griff with an amused grin and said, "I am the Carlens of the Carlens tube!" He invited Griff to come to see a mediastinoscopy. Although Carlens had published a paper in 1959 on its use in the evaluation of mediastinal lymph nodes, Griff was not familiar with the procedure. Carlens let Griff put his finger and then a mediastinoscope through a low midline cervical incision, which allowed access to the paratracheal and pretracheal lymph nodes for pathologic diagnosis. On his return to Toronto, Griff championed the use of mediastinoscopy in the staging of lung cancer throughout North America to prevent futile thoracotomies in patients with unresectable mediastinal lung cancer metastasis. With the help of Dr Bob Ginsberg, he formed the first surgical group in Toronto to participate and lead a North American cooperative group (The Lung Cancer Study Group). Ever since that time, the Toronto team has been a leader in clinical trials of lung and esophageal cancer treatment in North America.

In 1960, he returned to the TGH, where he quickly established himself as a thoughtful clinical surgeon and investigator. In 1967, he joined Dr Norman Delarue in starting the first Division of Thoracic Surgery in Canada. Griff's students called him "the Pied Piper of Thoracic Surgery." His cheerfulness, curiosity, sense of wonder, clear communication skills, and surgical agility attracted surgeons, physicians, and nurses from throughout the world to join the TGH thoracic team. Dr Pearson established a training program in Thoracic Surgery that was recognized by the Royal College of Physicians

Thorac Surg Clin 28 (2018) xiii–xiv
https://doi.org/10.1016/j.thorsurg.2018.02.005
1547-4127/18/© 2018 Published by Elsevier Inc.

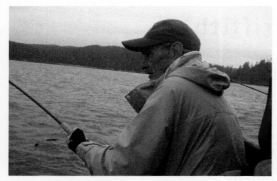

Fig. 1. Dr Frederick Griffith Pearson.

and Surgeons of Canada in 1977, as a separate specialty. This program has been a template for training programs throughout North America and the world. The majority of graduates of the "Toronto Program" are now leaders in the field of general thoracic surgery in Canada and throughout North and South America, Europe, and Asia.

Dr Pearson established the first research laboratory in Thoracic Surgery in Canada. The Thoracic Surgical Research Laboratories have made seminal contributions in airway surgery, lung transplantation, and lung oncology. In 1968, Pearson, Goldberg, and da Silva published "Tracheal stenosis complicating tracheostomy with cuffed tubes. Clinical experience and observations from a prospective study" (Arch Surg 1968;97(3):380–94). In 1971, Pearson and Andrews published "Detection and management of tracheal stenosis following cuffed tube tracheostomy" (Ann Thorac Surg 1971;12(4):359–74). Griff's close collaboration with Dr Hermes Grillo at the Massachusetts General Hospital led to the recruitment of Dr Joel Cooper to the TGH from Dr Grillo's thoracic program. In 1975, Pearson, Cooper, and Nelems described "Primary tracheal anastomosis after resection of cricoid cartilage with preservation of recurrent laryngeal nerves" (J Thorac Cardiovasc Surg 1975;70(5):806–16). This "Pearson technique" has proven to be very effective in the management of subglottic stenosis. Cooper and Pearson also described the "Use of silicone stents in the management of airway problems" (Ann Thorac Surg 1989;47(3):371–8).

Based on these research discoveries in the lab, the TGH lung transplant team of Joel Cooper, Bill Nelems, Tom Todd, Mel Goldberg, and Alex Patterson carried out the first successful lung transplant in the world in 1983. Under the leadership of Dr Shaf Keshavjee and Dr Tom Waddell, this group continues to innovate in lung transplantation and tissue regeneration and now carries out more than 120 lung transplants a year.

Always humble, he has been honored by being appointed as the Surgeon-in-Chief at the TGH, the President of the American Association of Thoracic Surgeons, a member of the Order of Canada, and an Honorary Fellow of five international thoracic societies. Griff was the lead editor of the first and second editions of the popular Pearson's textbook of thoracic and esophageal surgery. Recently, he coauthored *Evolution of Thoracic Surgery in Canada* with Dr Jean Deslauriers and Dr Bill Nelems.

Dr Pearson's greatest legacy was as a teacher and mentor. He had a clear understanding of the practice of thoracic surgery and all of its nuances. His ethics, teaching, and discoveries continue to influence thoracic surgeons around the world. Dr Frederick Griffith Pearson, aged 90, died in Kitchener on August 10, 2016 surrounded by his wife, Hilppa Pearson, and his family.

Richard J. Finley, MD, FRCSC, FACS
Emeritus Professor of Surgery
University of British Columbia
Vancouver, British Columbia V5Z 1M9, Canada

E-mail address:
richard.finley@vch.ca

General Considerations

Birth of Airway Surgery and Evolution over the Past Fifty Years

Jean Deslauriers, MD, FRCS(C), CM

KEYWORDS

- Airway surgery • History • Evolution of airway surgery

KEY POINTS

- Significant developments in airway surgery took place following the introduction of mechanical ventilators and intubation with cuffed endotracheal tubes during the worldwide epidemic of poliomyelitis in the early 1950s.
- In the early 1960s, it was generally accepted that surgeons could remove no more than 2 or 3 tracheal rings (2-cm rule) and predictably be able to reconstruct the airway.
- In the adult patient, about half the tracheal length can now be circumferentially resected and continuity restored by primary end-to-end anastomosis.
- The most prominent pioneers in airway surgery were Dr Frederick G Pearson from Toronto, Dr Hermes C Grillo from Boston, and Mr Louis Couraud from Bordeaux, France.

INTRODUCTION

Significant developments in airway surgery mainly took place following the introduction of mechanical ventilators and intubation with cuffed endotracheal or tracheostomy tubes during the worldwide epidemic of poliomyelitis in 1952. The first mechanical ventilators, which were simple volume units, were designed in Denmark. Meanwhile, Swedish engineers created the more sophisticated Engstrom Ventilator, which possessed both volume and pressure controls. By the late 1950s, these Engstrom units were in common use throughout Europe and North America. At the time, both the endotracheal and tracheostomy tubes were thick-walled and rigid, and the balloons were round and firm. The plethora of tracheal injuries that followed the use of such tubes provided surgeons with extensive experience with resection and reconstruction of secondary stenotic tracheal lesions.

In the early 1960s, it was generally accepted that surgeons could safely remove no more than a few centimeters of trachea because it was believed that tracheobronchial tissues healed poorly as compared with those of the stomach, intestine, and even skin.[1] It was also believed that both the rigidity and poor blood supply of the cartilaginous airway structure were major handicaps. Finally, it was thought that anesthesia could be difficult to maintain during airway reconstruction.

The most important contributors to the birth and evolution of airway surgery were Dr Frederick Griffith Griff Pearson from Toronto, Ontario, Canada (1926–2016) (**Fig. 1**); Dr Hermes C Grillo from Boston, Massachusetts, USA (1923–2003) (**Fig. 2**); and Mr Louis Couraud from Bordeaux, France (1929–2016) (**Fig. 3**). Other notable contributors were Professor Mikhail Perelman from Moscow in the Soviet Union and Mr Henry Eschapasse (1919-present) from Toulouse, France (**Fig. 4**).

Looking back is a respectful pursuit because it pays tribute to the heritage and pioneers (**Fig. 5**) of airway surgery while providing some insight into the roots and evolution of our profession in this field.

Disclosure: The author has nothing to disclose.
Laval University, 6364, Chemin Royal, Saint-Laurent-de-l'Île-d'Orléans, Quebec City, Quebec G0A3Z0, Canada
E-mail address: jean.deslauriers@chg.ulaval.ca

Thorac Surg Clin 28 (2018) 109–115
https://doi.org/10.1016/j.thorsurg.2018.02.001

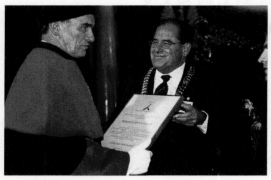

Fig. 1. Dr FG Pearson from Toronto, Ontario, Canada (*on the left*) receiving an award for his work on airway surgery from Professor Francisco (Paco) Paris Romeu from Valencia, Spain, President of the European Society of Thoracic Surgery.

PATHOGENESIS OF BENIGN TRACHEAL STRICTURES AND BIRTH OF AIRWAY SURGERY

Before the early 1970s, numerous factors were thought to be associated with the occurrence of benign tracheal strictures (**Box 1**) but its true etiologic origin remained a mystery. In 1968, Drs Griff Pearson and Melvyn Goldberg[2] from Toronto

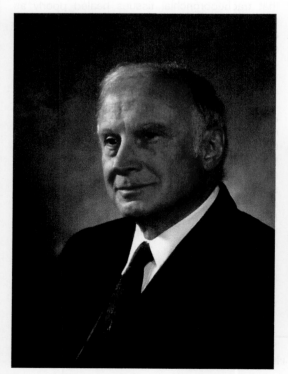

Fig. 2. Dr Hermes C Grillo from Boston, Massachusetts, USA, a true legend in airway surgery.

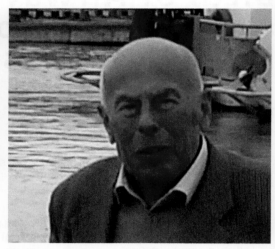

Fig. 3. Mr Louis Couraud from Bordeaux, France, a world expert in laryngotracheal surgery.

made the observation that high ventilator pressures (therefore, high pressure between the endotracheal tube cuff and tracheal wall) were likely the most important pathogenetic factors in the development of benign tracheal strictures. In this seminal paper, they wrote the following:

> In seven patients, stenosis developed in the mediastinal trachea at the level of the inflatable cuff. In each patient, the lesion was identified as a firm, concentric, fibrous stenosis. It is assumed that pressure between the cuff and the tracheal wall led to circumferential mucosal ulceration and injury to underlying connective tissue and cartilage with subsequent healing by concentric scar contracture.

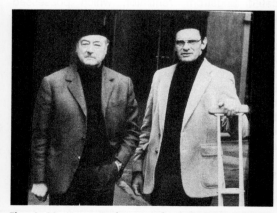

Fig. 4. Mr Henry Eschapasse from Toulouse, France (*left*), a world expert in airway neoplasms with Dr FG Pearson. The photograph was taken in 1981 before a meeting on tracheobronchial surgery held in Bordeaux.

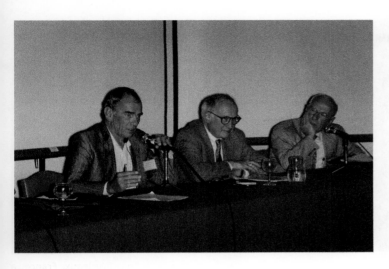

Fig. 5. The legendary so-called 3 Musketeers of airway surgery taken in Punta del Este, Uruguay in 1995. From left to right: Dr FG Pearson, Dr Hermes C Grillo, and Mr Louis Couraud.

In 1969, Dr Joel D Cooper, then a research fellow at the Massachusetts General Hospital in Boston, and Dr Hermes C Grillo experimentally produced erosive lesions of the trachea at the cuff site in dogs. These erosions occurred within 5 days to 2 weeks of inflating conventional tracheostomy tube cuffs at clinically used pressures.[3,4] They further showed that large-volume latex cuffs, with low intraluminal pressure, produced no significant lesions, either grossly or microscopically. The conclusion of these most important observations were that, Those two findings conclusively confirm clinical and pathological evidence that tracheal erosions and subsequent stenosis at the site of the tracheostomy tube cuff originate from pressure necrosis caused by the cuff.

Little work on segmental tracheal resection was done before the early 1960s, although the late Ronald Belsey[5] (**Fig. 6**) had reported as early as 1950 on 2 patients in whom adequate airways had been restored following resection of the

intrathoracic trachea. In that paper, Belsey wrote that the delays in developing surgery of the trachea could be attributed to 3 factors (**Box 2**). With his typical wisdom, Belsey added, "The intrathoracic portion of the trachea is the last unpaired organ in the body to fall to the surgeon, and the successful solution of the problem of its reconstruction may mark the end of the 'expansionist' epoch in the development of surgery."

In 1960, it was generally accepted that surgeons could safely remove no more than 2 or 3 tracheal rings, the so-called 2-cm rule, and predictably be able to reconstruct the airway with primary anastomosis. By the late 1960s, however, this 2-cm rule was being challenged owing to improved knowledge of airway anatomy and blood supply, better preoperative imaging techniques, use of tension-releasing maneuvers, and better anesthetic techniques. In the adult patient, for instance, more than half of the tracheal length can now be circumferentially removed and continuity restored by primary end-to-end anastomosis. As was originally reported in 1971 by Pearson and Andrews,[6] successful primary anastomosis depends on adequate resection of the diseased airway, mobilization of the trachea with preservation of maximal circulation, avoidance of anastomotic tension, and optimal anesthetic technique during reconstruction.

OPERATIVE CHALLENGE OF SUBGLOTTIC TRACHEAL RESECTION

When benign stenotic lesions involve the airway at the cricoid level, surgery becomes more complex because complete transection of the airway inevitably results in the division of both recurrent laryngeal nerves. For this reason, stenotic cricoid lesions were originally managed by repetitive

---

Box 1
Factors thought to be associated with benign tracheal strictures

- Cartilage does not regenerate
- Size and tip of the tracheostomy cannula
- Tight suturing of wound about the tracheotomy tube encourages peritracheal infection and perichondritis
- Hypoxia and altered tissue response to hypotension
- Duration of cannulation and type of incision

Data from Goldberg M, Pearson FG. Pathogenesis of tracheal stenosis following tracheostomy with a cuffed tube. Thorax 1972;27:678–91.

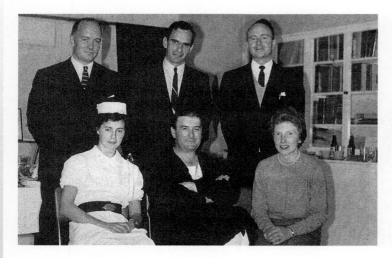

Fig. 6. Frenchay Hospital in Bristol, United Kingdom, 1959. Standing from left to right: Dr Charles Burns, who became the head of general surgery in Winnipeg, Manitoba, Canada; Dr FG Pearson; and Dr Bill Spence, who became a general surgeon at Toronto General Hospital. Sitting from left to right: Sister Steele, head nurse in Belsey's operating room; Ronald Belsey; and Peggie Spence, Spence's wife.

dilatations, staged plastic reconstructions, prolonged stenting, or permanent tracheostomies.

In 1975, Griff Pearson and colleagues,[7] from the Toronto General Hospital, reported on 6 patients with subglottic lesions involving the cricoid who had been treated by segmental resection and removal of all but a thin shell of posterior cricoid lamina, allowing for preservation of the recurrent laryngeal nerves (**Fig. 7**). The operation, now called the Pearson operation, is among the most significant contributions to airway surgery of all time. In a later publication, while a resident in thoracic surgery in Toronto, Dr Michael A Maddaus and colleagues[8] (FG Pearson) wrote, "We conclude that selected patients with benign stenosis involving both the glottis and subglottis may be successfully managed by synchronous correction of both lesions with good results. The collaboration of the Departments of Otolaryngology and Thoracic Surgery is essential to achieve those results."

In 1995, Mr Louis Couraud and colleagues[9] reported on a series of 217 nontumoral stenoses of

the upper airway, including 97 laryngotracheal stenosis, some of them involving the supraglottic and glottic regions that had been treated by surgery between 1978 and 1992. To this day, this series, along with the series of 502 cases by Hermes Grillo and colleagues,[10] remains among the largest ever reported on the issue. In his discussion of the presentation by Louis Couraud and colleagues,[9] Dr FG Pearson said, "I visited Dr Couraud in Bordeaux and know that he is a pragmatic, experienced clinician and an extremely skilled technical surgeon, and his observations are critical and original. He learns from his own observations, and has made some very original contributions, which have been presented here today."

SURGERY OF THE CARINA

Although there are relatively few indications for carinal resection and reconstruction, some tumors of the lower trachea or proximal main bronchi are amenable to surgery. In 1976, while a resident in Toronto, Dr Terry Theman and colleagues[11] (FG Pearson) reported on 2 cases in which they had used a pant leg reconstruction of the bronchial stumps, which was then anastomosed to the distal trachea. Both patients did well postoperatively, and the investigators concluded that there was seldom an indication for cardiopulmonary bypass in such cases because most could be managed by conventional techniques of intermittent ventilation with the appropriate tubes and sterile intraoperative connectors.

When lung cancer involves the carina, the tumor is usually so extensive that a curative resection is not possible. There are, however, occasional cases that are sufficiently localized to allow for complete resection and primary

---

Box 2
Factors that have delayed the surgical attack on the trachea

- As in the case of the heart, trachea function cannot be suspended, even temporarily
- The healing properties of the trachea have been suspect
- No satisfactory method of bypassing this organ (as in the bowel) has yet been described, and any resection must be followed by restoration of continuity

Data from Belsey R. Resection and reconstruction of the intrathoracic trachea. Br J Surg 1950;38:200–5.

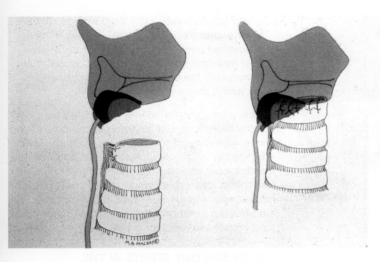

Fig. 7. The Pearson operation for subglottic strictures. The oblique resection line begins anteriorly at the inferior border of the thyroid cartilage and extends posteriorly through the lower border of the cricoid plate below the point of entry of the recurrent laryngeal nerves. (*From* Deslauriers J, Nelems B, Pearson, FG. Evolution of thoracic surgery in Canada. Hamilton (Canada): Decker Intellectual Properties; 2015; with permission.)

reconstruction. One of the first surgical attempts to deal with this problem was an operation described by Dr Frederick G Kergin[12] and now called the Kergin pneumonectomy. Interestingly, Dr Kergin had been the mentor of Griff Pearson at Toronto General Hospital. The gist of the Kergin pneumonectomy was the resection of the lesion along with the lateral portion of the trachea, carried down to the right main bronchus in such a way as to create a pedicle graft of the right main bronchus in continuity with the carina; when turned upward and tailored, this flap sealed the gap in the trachea (**Fig. 8**).

The alternative to the Kergin pneumonectomy is a full carinal pneumonectomy, first reported in 1959 by J. Maxwell Gibbon and colleagues.[13] It was subsequently popularized by Dr Bob Jensik and colleagues,[14] from Chicago in 1972, and Dr Jean Deslauriers and colleagues,[15] including Dr Maurice Beaulieu from Quebec City, Quebec, Canada in 1979.

FROM THE USE OF TRACHEAL PROSTHESIS TO TISSUE ENGINEERING

After tracheal resection, the airway can usually be primarily reconstructed with end-to-end anastomosis, although, on occasion, long segments of trachea have been removed, and the surgeon tempted to resort to the use of an interposed graft or prosthesis. Over the years, a great variety of solid prosthetic tubes have been used in both experimental and clinical settings but the results have generally been unsatisfactory.

In 1968, Griff Pearson and colleagues[16] reported the results of experimental and clinical studies on tracheal reconstruction with an interposed heavy porous Marlex mesh (**Fig. 9**). Epithelialization of the endoluminal surface of the prosthesis occurred from the cut ends of the trachea; however, there was a tendency to stenosis in the midportion of the prosthesis, presumably due to excessive proliferation of granulation tissue

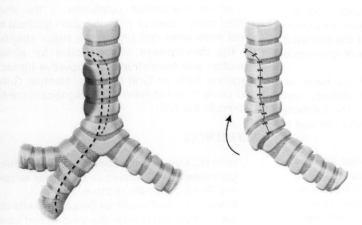

Fig. 8. Kergin pneumonectomy. Reconstruction of the trachea using a pedicle graft from the right main bronchus.

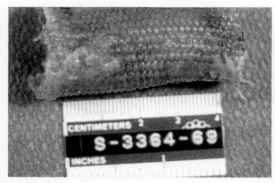

Fig. 9. Marlex mesh used by Griff Pearson in his experiments on bridging tracheal defects with a porous prosthesis.

in the part of the prosthesis that took longest to epithelialize.

In that same publication, Griff Pearson and colleagues[16] reported 2 successful clinical cases, both with adenoid cystic carcinomas, which had required extensive airway resection from the cricothyroid membrane to the lower half of the intrathoracic trachea and reconstruction with a Marlex prosthesis. Twenty-eight years later, while working as a thoracic surgeon in Ottawa but a resident at the time, Dr Donna Maziak and colleagues[17] reviewed the Toronto experience in 38 patients with adenoid cystic carcinoma of the upper airway treated between 1963 and 1995. One case in that series deserves mention because it illustrates in spectacular fashion the evolution of airway surgery throughout the years. The patient had first been operated on in 1963; the case was 1 of the 2 reported on in 1968 in which a Marlex prosthesis had been used for reconstruction.[16] Five years after the initial operation, the patient was again operated for a local recurrence. By using newly developed release maneuvers at the upper and lower ends of the airway, the prosthesis and tracheal ends could be removed and, this time, the airway could be reconstructed by primary anastomosis. The patient survived the operation only to die in 1992 of yet another local recurrence, 29 years after the original surgery.

Although episodic successes have been reported with a variety of foreign prostheses, most still founder on a biological reef.[18] The following is what Hermes C Grillo wrote about the use of tracheal prosthesis[17]:

> When foreign material is implanted into the body in contact with an epithelial margin, a chronic nonhealing ulcer results. The usual results are, after a time, obstruction due to chronic granulations or erosion of major

blood vessels with fatal hemorrhage. None of the prosthetics currently available have triumphed over these problems to a degree that makes them safe in general usage. It is particularly the case in the lengthy resections for which they are truly needed.

New concepts for airway reconstruction after lengthy resections include tracheal transplantation and engineering of the airway epithelium. Tissue engineering strategies promote and accelerate macroscopic and microscopic epithelial repair by controlling cell organization using chemical and mechanical signals. Both of these approaches are showing great promise and have the potential to abrogate the need for prosthesis.

USE OF SILICONE STENTS IN THE MANAGEMENT OF COMPLEX AIRWAY PROBLEMS

On occasion, complicated problems occur for which resection and anastomosis may be inadequate or inappropriate. In some of these complex cases, Dr Joel Cooper and colleagues[19] from Toronto (FG Pearson) have shown that the tracheal T-tube, originally described by Dr William Montgomery[20] in 1968, may be used as a stent for the upper airway, either as a sole procedure or as an adjunct to surgical resection.

The T-tube maintains the patency of the upper airway and, unlike a tracheostomy tube, is non-irritating, provides respiration through the nasopharynx so that normal humidification and phonation are preserved, and generally requires little (if any) cleaning or special maintenance.

SUMMARY

Before 1950, reports of segmental tracheal resection and reconstruction by primary anastomosis were rare and most were anecdotal. With the advent of mechanical ventilation in the early 1960s, many cases of postintubation tracheal injuries were seen and provided a major stimulus for the development of techniques for airway resection and reconstruction. Innovative thoracic surgeons such as Griff Pearson, Hermes Grillo, and Louis Couraud have made significant contributions in this field.

REFERENCES

1. Grillo HC. Development of tracheal surgery: a historical review. Part 1: techniques of tracheal surgery. Ann Thorac Surg 2003;75:610–9.
2. Pearson FG, Goldberg M, da Silva AJ. Tracheal stenosis complicating tracheostomy with cuffed tubes.

Clinical experience and observations from a prospective study. Arch Surg 1968;97:380–94.

3. Cooper JD, Grillo HC. Experimental production and prevention of injury due to cuffed tracheal tubes. Surg Gynecol Obstet 1969;129:1235–41.

4. Cooper JD, Grillo HC. The evolution of tracheal injury due to ventilatory assistance through cuffed tubes: a pathologic study. Ann Surg 1969;169:334–48.

5. Belsey R. Resection and reconstruction of the intrathoracic trachea. Br J Surg 1950;38:200–5.

6. Pearson FG, Andrews MJ. Detection and management of tracheal stenosis following cuffed tube tracheostomy. Ann Thorac Surg 1971;12:359–74.

7. Pearson FG, Cooper JD, Nelems JM, et al. Primary tracheal anastomosis after resection of the cricoid cartilage with preservation of recurrent laryngeal nerves. J Thorac Cardiovasc Surg 1975;70:806–16.

8. Maddaus MA, Toth JLR, Gullane PJ, et al. Subglottic tracheal resection and synchronous laryngeal reconstruction. J Thorac Cardiovasc Surg 1992; 104:1443–50.

9. Couraud L, Jougon JB, Velly JF. Surgical treatment of nontumoral stenosis of the upper airway. Ann Thorac Surg 1995;60:250–60 [discussion 259–60].

10. Grillo HC, Donahue DM, Mathisen DJ, et al. Post-intubation tracheal stenosis. Treatment and results. J Thorac Cardiovasc Surg 1995;109:486–93.

11. Theman TE, Kerr JH, Nelems JM, et al. Carinal resection. A report of two cases and a description of the anesthetic technique. J Thorac Cardiovasc Surg 1976;71:314–20.

12. Kergin FG. Carcinoma of the trachea. J Thorac Surg 1952;23:164–8.

13. Gibbon JH, Chamberlain JM, et al. Bronchogenic carcinoma. An aggressive surgical attitude. J Thorac Surg 1959;38:741.

14. Jensik RJ, Faber LP, Milloy FJ, et al. Tracheal sleeve pneumonectomy for advanced carcinoma of the lung. Surg Gynecol Obstet 1972;134:231–6.

15. Deslauriers J, Beaulieu M, Bénazéra A, et al. Sleeve pneumonectomy for bronchogenic carcinoma. Ann Thorac Surg 1979;28:465–74.

16. Pearson FG, Henderson RD, Gross AE, et al. The reconstruction of circumferential tracheal defects with a porous prosthesis. An experimental and clinical study using heavy marlex mesh. J Thorac Cardiovasc Surg 1968;55:605–16.

17. Maziak DE, Todd TRJ, Keshavjee SH, et al. Adenoid cystic carcinoma of the airway: thirty-two-year experience. J Thorac Cardiovasc Surg 1996;112: 1522–32.

18. Grillo HC. Notes on the windpipe. Ann Thorac Surg 1989;47:9–26.

19. Cooper JD, Todd TRJ, Ilves R, et al. Use of the silicone tracheal T-tube for the managament of complex tracheal injuries. J Thorac Cardiovasc Surg 1981;82:559–68.

20. Montgomery WW. The surgical management of supraglottic and subglottic stenosis. Ann Otol Rhinol Laryngol 1968;77:534–46.

Fundamental and Practical Aspects of Airway Anatomy
From Glottis to Segmental Bronchus

Reza J. Mehran, MDCM, MSc, FRCSC

KEYWORDS

- Trachea • Airway • Carina • Bronchi

KEY POINTS

- Half of the trachea is in the neck and the other half is in the posterior mediastinum.
- In the neck, the recurrent laryngeal nerves are at risk of injury.
- In the thoracic inlet, contact with the right brachiocephalic artery can lead to erosion if a tracheostomy is placed too low.
- Close contact to the azygos vein can lead to injury during a mediastinoscopy.
- The carina can be exposed via a midline or right thoracotomy approach.

INTRODUCTION

Surgical interventions involving the airways are complex, and complications arising from manipulations of the airways can often be life threatening. Understanding the anatomy is an essential component of a safe surgical outcome. The objective of this article is to review the anatomy of the major airways pertinent to the most common surgical procedures in or around the airways, such as resection of the trachea, mediastinoscopy, and sleeve resections.

FUNDAMENTALS OF TRACHEAL ANATOMY

The human trachea starts from below the vocal cords down to the carina, where it divides itself between 2 mainstem bronchi, which end in the hilum of each lung. The glottis is the space between the vocal cords that allows the passage of air in and out of the trachea via the contractions of the diaphragm and other accessory respiratory muscles.

The length of the trachea is 10 to 13 cm with a diameter of 4 mm at birth to about 23×18 mm at full growth. The formula of (age in years +16)/4 is used in the pediatric population to determine the size of the endotracheal tube to be used. In adults, another quick reference is to use the size of the index finger.[1]

The trachea is made of a cartilaginous support frame to prevent collapse during the negative pressures generated during the inspiratory cycle. There are 15 to 22 cartilages, each with a thickness of about 4 mm. The first tracheal cartilage is immediately below the cricoid cartilage, which is the only continuous ring.

The subglottic area is part of the larynx that is formed of the supraglottis, glottis, and subglottis. The subglottis consists of the space immediately below the true vocal cords. Anteriorly, it is bordered by the thyrocricoid membrane and posteriorly by the posterior aspect of the cricoid cartilage. The cricothyroid membrane is the site of insertion of a temporary emergency tracheostomy,

Disclosure: The author has nothing to disclose.
Department of Thoracic Surgery, University of Texas MD Anderson Cancer Center, 1400 Pressler Street, FCT 19.5062, Unit 1489, Houston, TX 77030-4009, USA
E-mail address: RJMehran@MDAnderson.org

Thorac Surg Clin 28 (2018) 117–125
https://doi.org/10.1016/j.thorsurg.2018.02.003
1547-4127/18/© 2018 Elsevier Inc. All rights reserved.

because it is easily palpable in all individuals and is relatively avascular and wide with the neck in hyperextension. The cricopharyngeous muscle inserts in part to the cricoid cartilage and forms the cricopharyngeal sphincter known also as the Killian sling. Posteriorly, the sling is bordered on its superior aspect by the Killian triangle and inferiorly the Laimer triangle, both sites of the formation of esophageal diverticula.

The recurrent nerve dives below the cricopharyngeus muscle, against the trachea and the cricoid cartilage to innervate the true vocal cords. The intimate anatomic position of the recurrent laryngeal nerves and the trachea must always be remembered during dissection of the trachea in the neck on both sides, and during the dissection of the left border of the trachea in the mediastinum.

The tracheal cartilages are horseshoe shaped. They become circumferential at the level of the segmental bronchi. The vocal cord and the membranous portion of the trachea help with the creation of auto-PEEP during a Valsalva maneuver or coughing.

The cartilages calcify with age, which makes them more friable during the insertion of sutures. Half of the tracheal length is in the neck and starts at the level of C6-7. The other half lies in the posterior mediastinum, where the trachea dives posteriorly in contact with the vertebral bodies down to the level of T4-5. The angle between the sternum and the trachea increases with age as the kyphosis of the thoracic spine becomes more pronounced, making a dissection of the carina in the elderly even more difficult through a midline approach (**Fig. 2**).

The trachea moves with the position of the neck, and the dissection of any part of the trachea in the neck or the upper thoracic trachea is eased by positioning the head of the patient in hyperextension if safe. The hyperextension is then reversed to remove tension on an anastomosis.

The origin of the blood supply for the cervical trachea is mainly the inferior thyroid artery, and in the chest, the intercostal arteries.[1] The blood supply of the trachea enters the trachea laterally at positions 3 and 9 o'clock. The position of the blood supply must be remembered during the dissection around the trachea. At the carina, the blood supply enters directly into the carina, and it is often injured during the dissection of station 7. That is why this station is always biopsied last, after nodes in stations 4R and 4L are sampled.

Because the blood supply of the trachea is segmental, in order to preserve that blood supply and prevent ischemia, lateral dissection of the trachea below the entry point of the vessels must be avoided. Limiting the dissection anterior to the position of entry of the blood supply during a mediastinoscopy will also limit bleeding during the procedure (**Fig. 3**).

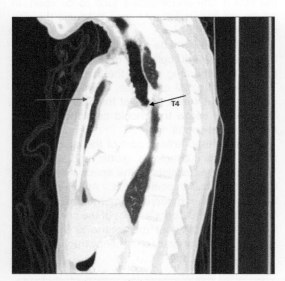

Fig. 1. Coronal view of the computed tomographic (CT) scan of a 40-year-old woman. Note the posterior deflection of the intrathoracic trachea. Note also that the carina (*black arrow*) lies just below the level of the angle of Louis (*red arrow*), the site of insertion of the cartilage of the second rib.

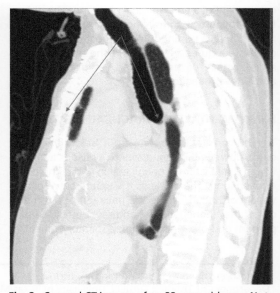

Fig. 2. Coronal CT images of an 82-year-old man. Note that the angle between the trachea (*red arrow*) and the sternum (*blue arrow*) is more pronounced than the younger patient in **Fig. 1**.

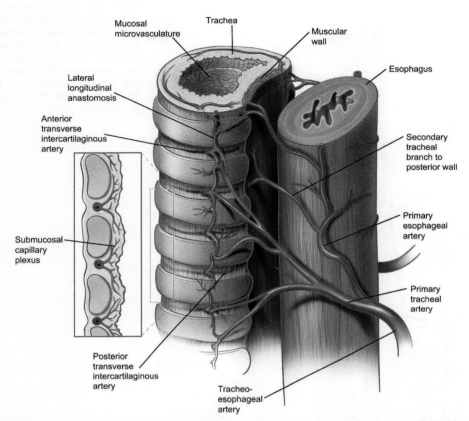

Mucosal microvasculature

Trachea

Muscular wall

Esophagus

Lateral longitudinal anastomosis

Anterior transverse intercartilaginous artery

Secondary tracheal branch to posterior wall

Submucosal capillary plexus

Primary esophageal artery

Primary tracheal artery

Posterior transverse intercartilaginous artery

Tracheo-esophageal artery

Fig. 3. Schematic presentation of the blood supply of the trachea. Note the lateral entry of the blood supply, which must be preserved during the dissection of the trachea. (*From* Minnich DJ, Mathisen DJ. Anatomy of the trachea, carina, and bronchi. Thorac Surg Clin 2007;17:578; with permission.)

SURGICAL ANATOMY OF THE CERVICAL TRACHEA

Whether a tracheostomy is performed by an open or percutaneous method, the cannula needs to be inserted at the level of the second or third tracheal rings, not below and not higher. Below that level, the cannula can come too close to the right brachiocephalic artery (**Figs. 4** and **5**). Above that level, the risk of tracheal stenosis increases. When performed open, the isthmus of the thyroid often needs to be divided.

Cervical tracheal resection is performed for tumor or mainly postintubation scarring. The most important structures to avoid during the circumferential dissection of the trachea are the recurrent laryngeal nerves. The dissection of the portion of the trachea to be resected must be done right against the trachea as so well illustrated by Dr Griff Pearson,[2] avoiding meandering in the area occupied by the recurrent nerve. The use of a bipolar cautery is essential. About 4 cm of the trachea can be removed, which is the equivalent of about 8 rings. The longer the segment of trachea to be resected is, the more the mediastinal trachea

needs to be freed from the surrounding structures. Anteriorly, the mobilization is achieved by dissecting the airway bluntly from the middle mediastinal vessels. Posteriorly, the trachea-esophageal fibroelastic membrane requires division. Sparse muscular fibers can be found in this area, which forms the residua of the trachea-esophageal septum (**Fig. 6**). The use of thermal energy devices can cause ischemic injuries to the membranous portion of the trachea, which is much thinner than the wall of the esophagus. As mentioned earlier, dissection of the lateral wall of the trachea is avoided to preserve the segmental blood supply.

THE MEDIASTINAL TRACHEA

The upper mediastinal trachea is best exposed through a midline sternotomy approach. The sternotomy can be partial with a transverse division of the sternum at or below the sternomanubrial junction, also known as the angle of Louis. The right brachiocephalic artery needs to be looped and dissected away from the trachea. If the tracheal repair falls posterior to the artery, the freshly

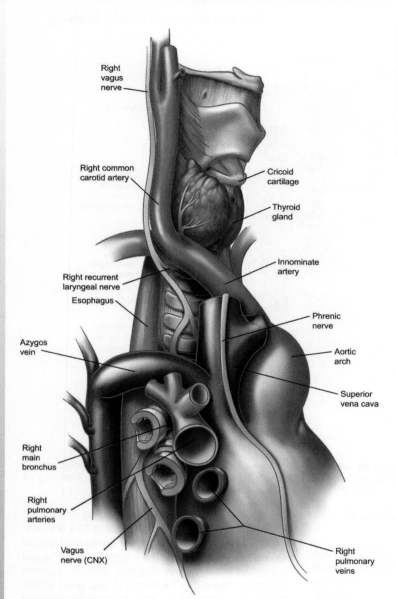

Fig. 4. Cervical and thoracic trachea. Note for the cervical trachea the position for the right brachiocephalic (innominate) artery, the thyroid gland, and both recurrent laryngeal nerves. (*From* Minnich DJ, Mathisen DJ. Anatomy of the trachea, carina, and bronchi. Thorac Surg Clin 2007;17:579; with permission.)

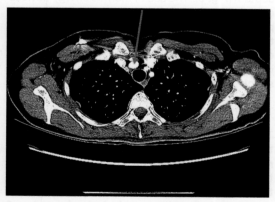

Fig. 5. The anatomy of the trachea at the thoracic inlet. Note the contact with the right brachiocephalic artery (*arrow*).

repaired trachea must be separated from the artery with a pedicle of vascularized tissue, such as with a pedicle of thymus to prevent future development of a tracheovascular (innominate) fistula.

Mediastinoscopy, although a simple procedure, can rapidly become very complicated if a vascular injury occurs. The most common vessel injured is the azygos vein just proximal to its insertion to the vena cava (**Figs. 7** and **8**). The other structure at risk is the left recurrent laryngeal nerve, when the nerve loops around the arch of the aorta and travels upward along the left lateral border of the trachea. In that location, the nerve can easily be injured by sampling of a mediastinal lymph node

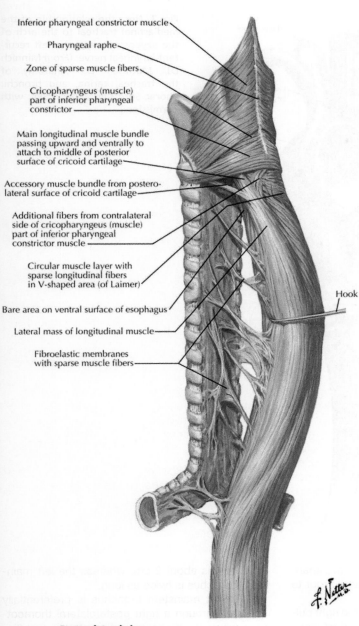

Inferior pharyngeal constrictor muscle

Pharyngeal raphe

Zone of sparse muscle fibers

Cricopharyngeus (muscle) part of inferior pharyngeal constrictor

Main longitudinal muscle bundle passing upward and ventrally to attach to middle of posterior surface of cricoid cartilage

Accessory muscle bundle from postero-lateral surface of cricoid cartilage

Additional fibers from contralateral side of cricopharyngeus (muscle) part of inferior pharyngeal constrictor muscle

Circular muscle layer with sparse longitudinal fibers in V-shaped area (of Laimer)

Bare area on ventral surface of esophagus

Lateral mass of longitudinal muscle

Fibroelastic membranes with sparse muscle fibers

Hook

Fig. 6. The anatomy of the tracheoesophageal space. Note the fibroelastic and muscular fibers between the trachea and esophagus, the remnants of the fetal tracheoesophageal septum and membrane. (*From* Netter FH. Musculature of esophagus, plate 231. In: Atlas of human anatomy. 6th edition. Philadelphia: Saunders/Elsevier; 2014; with permission.)

Posterolateral view

station 4L.[3] Permanent injury occurs in about 0.6% of mediastinoscopies, and this risk must be part of the informed consent. Transient injuries are thought to be much more frequent and could be a factor in the development of postoperative pneumonia after thoracic surgery done concomitantly.[4]

Resection of the trachea below the brachiocephalic artery, or resection of the carina, will need exposure of the entire posterior mediastinal trachea. The approach is best gained through the midline with a complete sternal division or through the right chest via a right posterolateral thoracotomy.

Through a midline approach, the trachea is exposed after opening of the anterior and posterior pericardium between the aorta and the superior vena cava, through the superior and the right pulmonary artery pericardial recesses (**Fig. 9**). The exposure is best maintained with a blunt instrument, such as the finger of the assistant on a sponge or with a malleable self-retaining retractor,

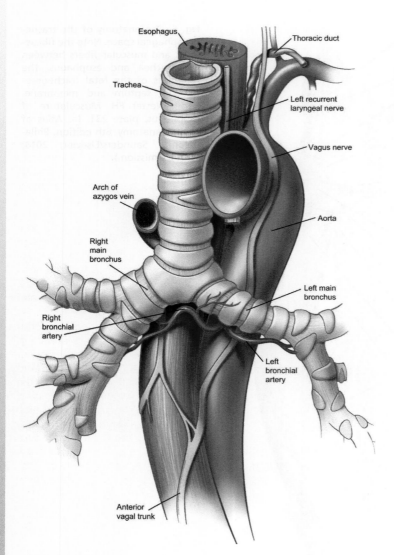

Esophagus

Thoracic duct

Trachea

Left recurrent
laryngeal nerve

Vagus nerve

Arch of
azygos vein

Aorta

Right
main
bronchus

Left main
bronchus

Right
bronchial
artery

Left
bronchial
artery

Anterior
vagal trunk

Fig. 7. Note the relationship of the mediastinal tracheal to the arch of the azygos vein and the left recurrent laryngeal nerve. (*From* Minnich DJ, Mathisen DJ. Anatomy of the trachea, carina, and bronchi. Thorac Surg Clin 2007;17:584; with permission.)

holding the aorta and the superior vena cava apart. Care must be taken with a calcified aortic root to prevent plaque embolization.

To gain better access to the carina, the right pulmonary artery may need to be retracted inferiorly with a vessel loop. This retraction may limit the blood flow through the artery, which can cause oxygenation issues if the procedure is combined with a right-sided ventilation, such as is the case during a left carinal pneumonectomy or left mainstem bronchus resection.

THE MAINSTEM BRONCHI

The right mainstem bronchus is more in line with the direction of the trachea, which makes the bronchus a more common site for foreign body impaction and aspiration. The length of the right mainstem is about 2 cm, whereas the left mainstem bronchus is twice as long.[5]

The right mainstem bronchus is preferentially exposed through a right posterolateral thoracotomy, where the bronchus is dissected by first flipping the lung anteriorly and then opening of the reflection of the parietal to visceral pleura. The proximal mainstem bronchus at the carina is better exposed by division of the azygos vein, which contacts the mainstem bronchus superiorly. This exposure can be continued distally to expose the right upper lobe bronchus and the bronchus intermedius. The pulmonary artery lies anterior to the right upper lobe bronchus and needs to be dissected away from the bronchus to facilitate a sleeve resection.

The entire left mainstem bronchus is well exposed through the midline as described earlier

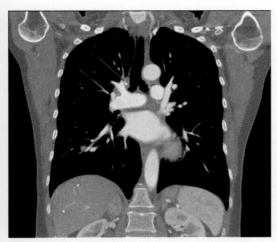

Fig. 8. Note the proximity of the azygos vein arch (*arrow*) to the right lateral wall of the mediastinal trachea just above the carina, in the lymph node station 4R territory.

and is a better option for cross-field ventilation than the right posterolateral thoracotomy approach. The left mainstem bronchus lies anterior to the esophagus. As mentioned before, the membranous portion of the left mainstem bronchus can easily be damaged by thermal dissection of the esophageal fibromuscular attachments (see **Fig. 6**).

LOBAR AND SEGMENTAL BRONCHI OF THE RIGHT LUNG

The right lung has 3 lobes: upper, middle, and lower. The right upper lobe bronchus, formally called the "eparterial bronchus," originates at a right angle from the right main bronchus

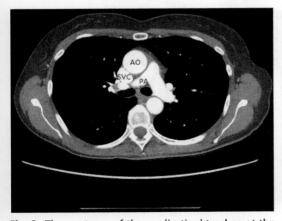

Fig. 9. The anatomy of the mediastinal trachea at the level of the carina. Note that a midline exposure will require an approach gained between the aorta (AO) and the superior vena cava (SVC). If necessary, the right pulmonary artery (PA) can be retracted inferiorly to gain access to the mainstem bronchi.

approximately 1.5 to 2.0 cm distal to the carina.[6] It is 1 cm long before dividing into 3 segmental bronchi supplying the apical (B1), the anterior (B2), and the posterior (B3) segments, respectively. It is smaller than its left counterpart, and it has a costovertebral external surface related to the curvature of the ribs and to the spine, a mediastinal internal surface, and a lower fissural surface. The origin of the right upper lobe bronchus often is anomalous in 3% of normal people, and the most common of such anomalies is that of the apical segmental bronchus of the right upper lobe bronchus originating directly from the right lateral wall of the trachea or right main bronchus.[7]

Proceeding distally from the takeoff of the right upper lobe, the right primary bronchus is called the "bronchus intermedius," which has a total length of 1.5 to 2.0 cm. It then gives rise anteriorly to the middle lobe bronchus, which divides into 2 segmental bronchi supplying the lateral (B4) and medial (B5) segments.

The right lower lobe lies inferior and posterior to the oblique fissure. The first segmental branch of the right lower lobe bronchus, the superior segmental (apical) bronchus (B6), originates from its posterior wall slightly distal to the origin of the middle lobe bronchus. The middle lobe bronchus and right lower lobe bronchus form the termination of the bronchus intermedius. The basal stem bronchus sends off 4 basal segmental bronchi to supply 4 basal segments, which are the medial basal segment (B7), the anterior basal segment (B8), the lateral basal segment (B9), and the posterior basal segment (B10).

LOBAR AND SEGMENTAL BRONCHI OF THE LEFT LUNG

The left lung has 2 lobes: upper and lower. It is made of 8 segments (vs 10 on the right side) because of sharing of the segmental bronchi by subsegmental bronchopulmonary units, which in the right lung are considered to be individual segments.

The left upper lobe bronchus arises anterolaterally from the main bronchus at a distance of approximately 4 to 5 cm from the carina. It bifurcates almost immediately into a superior trunk (culmen), which subdivides into an anterior segmental bronchus (B2) and a much larger common trunk for the apicoposterior segment (B1 and B3), and an inferior trunk forming the lingular orifice, which gives rise to the superior (B4) and inferior (B5) lingular bronchopulmonary segments.

The left lower lobe bronchus is the termination of the left main bronchus, and its general topographic anatomy is similar to that on the right side. At about half a centimeter from its origin, it gives rise posteriorly and laterally to the first segmental bronchus (superior segmental bronchus, B6). More distally (distance of 1.5 cm), the basal trunk gives rise to the anteromedial (B7 and B8), lateral basal (B9), and posterior basal (B10) segments. Contrary to the anatomy of the right lower lobe, the anterior and medial segments originate from a single branch of the lower lobe bronchus and are thus considered to be only one segment.

VASCULAR SUPPLY AND LYMPHATIC DRAINAGE OF BRONCHOPULMONARY SEGMENTS

One main segmental vein drains each bronchopulmonary segment, but contrary to the artery and bronchus, this vein runs in the intersegmental planes and thus marks the boundaries of each individual segment. Appreciation of this particularity of the venous drainage is a key to

the clinical application of anatomic segmentectomies or sleeve segmental resections.

The drainage pathway of pulmonary lymphatics is from subpleural vessels to larger channels running along segmental arteries and bronchi. Eventually, these lymphatics drain into subsegmental and segmental nodal stations.

The main indication of a segmental resection of the bronchus is the removal of a small tumor, most often a neuroendocrine carcinoma located at the takeoff of a segmental bronchus. The resection usually encompasses the segmental bronchus and the segment itself, and the residual segmental bronchus of that lobe is then sutured to the bronchus of the lobe. The main anatomic relationship to keep in mind during the dissection of the segmental bronchus is its close relationship to the segmental pulmonary artery, which always lies anterior and superior to the segmental bronchus (**Fig. 10**).

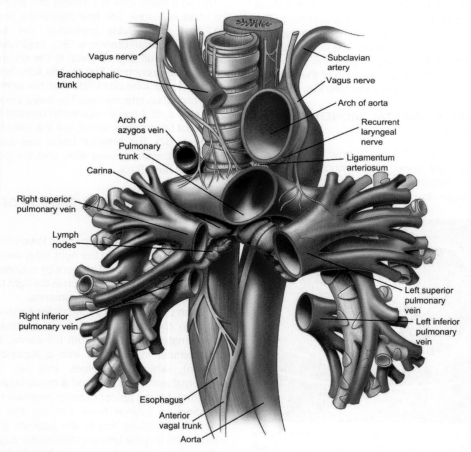

Fig. 10. Segmental anatomy of the airways. Note the intimate contact between segmental airways with the pulmonary artery. Segmental bronchoplasties are accomplished by dividing the segmental bronchus and a sleeve of the lobar bronchus intermedius and then approximation of the residual airways. (*From* Minnich DJ, Mathisen DJ. Anatomy of the trachea, carina, and bronchi. Thorac Surg Clin 2007;17:584; with permission.)

SUMMARY

Proper knowledge of the anatomy allows the surgeon to understand imaging, and as a result, the geography of the pathologic processes. This allows the surgeon to plan the roadmap to a cure. Attempts to perform airway procedures without the precise knowledge of the anatomy can only result in stressful procedures, with often less than optimal oncologic outcomes or vascular catastrophes. The mastery of anatomy insures that each patient is offered the best surgical resection for the condition they present with.

REFERENCES

1. Allen MS. Surgical anatomy of the trachea. Chest Surg Clin N Am 2003;13:191–9.

2. Maddaus MA, Toth JL, Gullane PJ, et al. Subglottic tracheal resection and synchronous laryngeal reconstruction. J Thorac Cardiovasc Surg 1992;104(5): 1443–50.

3. Minnich DJ, Mathisen DJ. Anatomy of the trachea, carina, and bronchi. Thorac Surg Clin 2007;17:571–85.

4. Lemaire A, Nikolic I, Petersen T, et al. Nine-year single center experience with cervical mediastinoscopy: complications and false negative rate. Ann Thorac Surg 2006;82(4):1185–9.

5. Drevet G, Conti M, Deslauriers J. Surgical anatomy of the tracheobronchial tree. J Thorac Dis 2016;8:S121–9.

6. Ugalde P, Camargo JDJ, Deslauriers J. Lobes, fissures, and bronchopulmonary segments. Thorac Surg Clin 2007;17:587–99.

7. Le Roux BT. Anatomical abnormalities of the right upper lobe bronchus. J Thorac Cardiovasc Surg 1962; 44:225–7.

Advanced Technologies for Imaging and Visualization of the Tracheobronchial Tree
From Computed Tomography and MRI to Virtual Endoscopy

Micheal C. McInnis, MD[a,b], Gordon Weisbrod, MD[b,c], Heidi Schmidt, MD[b,d],*

KEYWORDS

- Trachea • Computed tomography • MRI • Virtual endoscopy • Dynamic CT • Tracheal stenosis

KEY POINTS

- Virtual endoscopy plays a complementary role to flexible bronchoscopy and has a role to play in overcoming some inherent limitations of flexible bronchoscopy.
- Because of the significant advances in imaging, computed tomography can now provide accurate 3-dimensional reconstructions of the trachea.
- Imaging of the trachea assists in planning for bronchoscopy and surgical intervention.
- Dynamic expiratory imaging of the trachea is accurate in the diagnosis of tracheomalacia and superior to end-expiratory imaging.
- MRI is useful for imaging of vascular rings and may see increasing use in the pediatric patient population.

HISTORY

Imaging of the trachea has undergone a revolution over the course of Dr Pearson's career. Before computed tomography (CT), imaging of the trachea involved assessment by plain radiograph and tomography. Used over decades, these limited techniques did identify a few classic signs of disease, such as the saber-sheath trachea or steeple sign.[1,2] Given the early limitations of imaging, bronchoscopy has been long considered the gold standard for evaluation of the airway and is clearly superior to plain radiographic techniques. Other advances followed, such as bronchography, providing further insight into the radiographic appearance of the airways but remained of limited use until the advent of CT. Since then, there has been a continuous evolution with advances in

Disclosure: The authors have nothing to disclose.
[a] Joint Department of Medical Imaging, University Health Network, Mount Sinai Hospital, Women's College Hospital, 76 Grenville Street, Room 2248, Toronto, Ontario M5S 1B2, Canada; [b] Department of Medical Imaging, University of Toronto, 263 McCaul Street, Toronto, ON M5T 1W, Canada; [c] Joint Department of Medical Imaging, University Health Network, Mount Sinai Hospital, Women's College Hospital, Toronto General Hospital, 200 Elizabeth Street, Toronto, Ontario M5G 2C4, Canada; [d] Joint Department of Medical Imaging, University Health Network, Mount Sinai Hospital, Women's College Hospital, 76 Grenville Street, Room 2231, Toronto, Ontario M5S 1B2, Canada
* Corresponding author. Joint Department of Medical Imaging, Women's College Hospital, 76 Grenville Street, Room 2231, Toronto, Ontario M5S 1B2.
E-mail address: Heidi.Schmidt@uhn.ca

Thorac Surg Clin 28 (2018) 127–137
https://doi.org/10.1016/j.thorsurg.2018.01.005
1547-4127/18/© 2018 Elsevier Inc. All rights reserved.

computing power facilitating virtual endoscopy (VE) and entirely new methods, such as MRI of the airways. Although bronchoscopy is still regarded as the gold standard, advanced technologies for imaging of the airways have an important role to play where bronchoscopy meets limitations and in this way plays a complementary role. Some limitations of bronchoscopy overcome by imaging include the risks related to the invasiveness of the procedure, its inability to visualize structures external to the airway, as in the case with extrinsic compression, adjacent vasculature, or invasive tumors, as well as the inability to visualize distal to an obstruction.

COMPUTED TOMOGRAPHY
Technical Factors and Protocol

Multi-detector CT (MDCT) imaging of the trachea is preferably performed with 64 slices or greater. State-of-the-art CT tracheal imaging optimally uses up to 320 slices that span over a length of 16 cm. Generally, this would cover the length of the trachea and the scan could be completed in the time it takes for the CT gantry to make one complete rotation. This rapid rotation time reduces motion artifact inherent in imaging of the airways.

Detector collimation is narrow (1 mm or less) for high resolution and facilitating reformat reconstruction. The authors' standard protocol uses a tube current of 50 mA and tube voltage of 120 kV. The gantry rotation time is 0.5 seconds. Because a 320-slice CT can cover the length of the trachea in one rotation, the scan time will be equal to the gantry rotation time, thus, achieving very short scan times. Because the scan time is so short, the technique can be applied to patients with limited ability to breath-hold, including children and infants. The total radiation dose depends on patient factors and technical parameters but is less than a full chest CT. Low-dose techniques can be applied to adults when warranted and when imaging children.

Patients are instructed to cough before the procedure to clear secretions and positioned supine on the gantry table. Adequate patient instruction is critical for high-quality imaging with breathing instructions provided in the patients' preferred language. The scan is performed under breath-hold at full inspiration. Imaging of the trachea alone includes a narrow field of view of around 10 cm for optimal spatial resolution beginning from above the vocal cords to below the carina. This view excludes most of the lung. The entire chest may be scanned separately following the tracheal CT with a wide field of view to visualize the lungs and small airways. Studies are generally performed without contrast. Indications for intravenous contrast commonly include evaluation of tumors or vascular anatomy adjacent the trachea.

The authors routinely reconstruct their images in 3-mm-thick axial (transverse plane) slices with 1-mm or thinner slices available for review when needed. Images are reconstructed in a soft tissue kernel and an edge-enhanced (lung) kernel. Images are interpreted in lung windows to evaluate the lumen (window level, −600 Hounsfield units [HU]; window width, 1500 HU). Soft tissue windows (window level, 40 HU; window width, 350 HU) may be helpful for evaluating the tracheal wall and adjacent fat and identifying calcification.

Multi-planar Reformats

With the advent of helical CT and isotropic imaging, it is possible to reconstruct images in any desired plane, in 2 dimensions. Standard reconstructions for the trachea include axial, sagittal, and coronal planes; these are routinely performed on all scans. However, multi-planar reformats (MPRs) in oblique planes may be obtained particularly to display findings to the best advantage in a single image along the course of the entire trachea. Interpretation is routinely performed using the axial images, correlating with MPRs when necessary.

Three-Dimensional Volume-Rendered Images

Volume rendering provides bronchogramlike images of the tracheobronchial tree using postprocessing techniques.[3] The use of volume-rendered images, even on 16-slice CT scanners, has been shown to improve interpreter confidence, provide additional diagnostic information, and improve confidence in the interpretation of congenital airway abnormalities when compared with axial slices alone.[4] Volume rendering includes shaded surface display (SSD) as well as minimum intensity projection (MinIP) and maximum intensity projection (MIP) reconstructions. MinIP accentuates the air spaces and may be useful for demonstrating the tracheal air column. MIP has limited value in routine imaging of the trachea but does accentuate nodularity and filling defects.

SSD requires more operator manipulation but ultimately provides visually pleasing 3-dimensional (3D) reconstructions of the trachea that are of particular interest to the consulting physicians, as the presentation more closely mimics surgical anatomy than axial images alone.

Normal Computed Tomography Appearance

Although the detailed tracheal anatomy is familiar to the thoracic surgeon, there are key points to review as it pertains to the appearance on cross-sectional imaging. The normal trachea extends over a length of 10 to 12 cm and is demonstrated over its entire length on coronal or sagittal reformats. The width of the adult trachea is generally 2.0 to 2.5 cm with maximal cross-sectional areas reported in the literature.[5] The normal shape of the trachea on axial images of an inspiratory CT has been described most commonly as round, oval, or horseshoe-shaped with a flat posterior membrane.[5,6] The trachea may have a different shape at different levels.[6] The shape is attributed to cartilaginous anterior C-shaped rings, numbering 16 to 20 in total, with a flexible thin membranous posterior wall that moves with respiration. The tracheal wall is normally smooth aside from the undulations of cartilaginous rings. Thickening or nodularity may be a sign of disease but most commonly relates to retained secretions, a common imaging pitfall in evaluating the trachea.[7]

Computed Tomography Applications

Calcification

CT is useful for identifying airway calcifications. Diffuse calcification is not uncommon in elderly patients, referred to as senescent calcification, and more prevalent in women than in men. Diffuse calcification sparing the posterior membrane may also be seen in patients on long-term warfarin therapy.[8]

Calcification is an important indicator of disease when focal or nodular. Calcifications are seen in diseases, such as tracheobronchopathia osteochondroplastica (TPO), tracheobronchial amyloidosis (**Fig. 1**), and relapsing polychondritis.[9,10] Calcification can also be seen in masses, such as hamartomas, chondromas, and carcinoid tumors.

Tracheal stenosis

MDCT allows for accurate measurement of stenosis grade, length, length from vocal cord, and preoperative resection planning. Findings correlate well with the gold standard of preoperative bronchoscopy and intraoperative findings.[11,12] Although MDCT is highly accurate in identifying airway stenosis, there is a tendency to overestimate the true grade of stenosis.[13] Coronal or oblique coronal planes may display the entire length of the trachea, including the stenosis, in one image and is a helpful reference for referring physicians. MinIP reconstructions further accentuate the contrast between the stenosed airway lumen and the adjacent tracheal wall (**Fig. 2**).

The most common cause of tracheal narrowing is a saber-sheath trachea as seen in patients with chronic obstructive pulmonary disease (COPD) characterized by a narrowing of coronal diameter.[1] The most common cause of true stenosis relates to intubation; however, tracheal stenosis can also be seen as the sequela of a host of infectious and inflammatory processes. Apart from demonstrating the stenosis, CT may provide a clue as to the cause by revealing associated

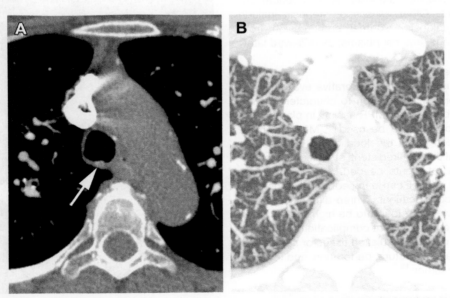

Fig. 1. (*A*) Axial CT in a 67-year-old woman with amyloidosis demonstrates a small calcified nodule (*arrow*) along the posterior wall of the trachea. (*B*) MIP image in the same patient accentuates tracheal irregularity seen cranial to the nodule in (*A*).

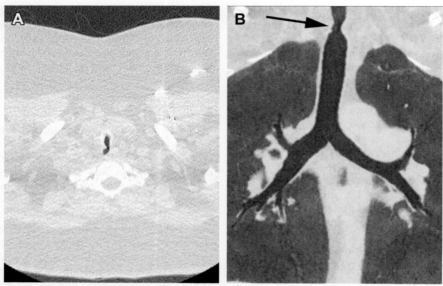

Fig. 2. (*A*) Axial CT image of a 44-year-old woman demonstrates a postintubation tracheal stenosis. (*B*) Coronal MinIP demonstrates the location of the stenosis in relation to the rest of the trachea (*arrow*). MinIP underestimates the degree of this stenosis.

disease findings. A classic inflammatory example is Wegener granulomatosis whereby in a small MDCT series of 10 patients all were found to have stenosis, 90% of the lesions being subglottic (**Fig. 3**).[14] Other inflammatory causes of stenosis demonstrated by CT are not common, such as inflammatory bowel disease, Behçet syndrome, and relapsing polychondritis.[15] Infection is reviewed more completely later, but a classic example of infection causing stenosis is *Mycobacterium tuberculosis*. Other causes of stenosis include TPO, amyloidosis, external compression from vascular rings, and neoplasms, as reviewed later.

Airway stents

MDCT is useful in the preoperative evaluation for airway stenting. In addition to characterizing the lesions to be stented, MPR assists in planning for the type of stent to be used.[16] MDCT can be used to determine the location of obstruction, diameter of the required stent, stent length, and total number of stents needed.[17] Following stent placement, MDCT can be used in monitoring the stent for complications. Three-dimensional renderings have been found to be highly accurate in the identification of stent complications, including narrowing due to granulation tissue or secretions, stent migration, fracture, perforation, and invasion of stent by tumor.[18]

Benign and malignant airway tumors

MDCT is complementary to bronchoscopy in the evaluation of tumors and is commonly performed

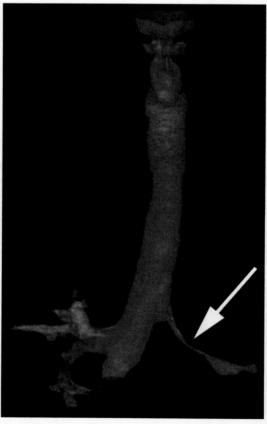

Fig. 3. Surface shade display in a 25-year-old man with granulomatosis with polyangiitis demonstrates a severe stenosis of the left main bronchus (*arrow*).

as a noninvasive first step. MDCT may be helpful in planning for biopsy of the tumor or suspicious lymph nodes. MDCT not only identifies a tumor within the airway but also details the extent of a tumor outside the airway within the mediastinum. There are limitations in that MDCT is insensitive in the detection of small mucosal-based lesions and retained airway secretions can be mistaken for pathology.[7,19] Malignant tumors of the trachea include squamous cell carcinoma, adenoid cystic carcinoma, mucoepidermoid carcinoma, carcinoid tumor, metastases (including direct invasion), and rare entities, such as primary sarcomas of the trachea and lymphoma (**Fig. 4**). Benign tumors include harmatoma, tracheobronchial papillomatosis, lipoma, leiomyoma, neurogenic tumors, and other rare entities.[20]

Infection

The trachea may be involved by acute or chronic viral, bacterial, and fungal infections. Infections of the trachea are most commonly viral, such as parainfluenza or respiratory syncytial virus, manifesting as focal or diffuse thickening (**Fig. 5**). On a frontal plain radiograph, infection of the large airways manifests as a steeple sign characterized by narrowing of the subglottic upper airway in pediatric patients with croup producing an inverted V shape.[2]

M tuberculosis of the tracheobronchial tree is less common in the era of modern medicine. In one study using CT with multi-planar and 3D volume-rendered images in patients with actively caseating disease, disease manifested as circumferential wall thickening, irregular luminal narrowing, and findings of mediastinitis.[21] When chronic and fibrotic, the infection manifests as fibrosis causing smooth, irregular, or occlusive airway disease.[21]

Fungal infection can involve the trachea, but there is limited literature on its appearance. In one series of patients with airway-invasive aspergillosis, disease in the trachea or main stem bronchi had no apparent imaging manifestations on MDCT in their 2 patients.[22] Immunosuppressed patients who have undergone a lung transplant are a cohort susceptible to aspergillus infection an airway at the bronchial anastomosis where tissue is relatively devascularized. Aspergillus can manifest as narrowing or stricture causing clinically relevant obstruction.[23]

Chronic tracheal infection can be seen in tracheobronchial papillomatosis caused by human papillomavirus. This infection is usually acquired at birth and manifests as endobronchial papillomas causing small endobronchial nodules or diffuse nodular thickening.[20] Rhinoscleroma, a chronic granulomatous infection extending from the nasopharynx to occasionally involve the trachea, causes tracheal stenosis; but imaging reports are sparse.[15]

Airway dilation and diverticula

CT readily demonstrates congenital tracheobronchomegaly (Mounier-Kuhn syndrome), which

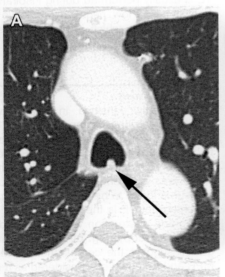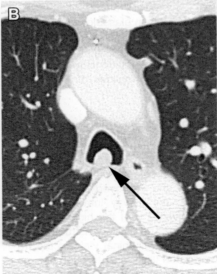

Fig. 4. (A) Axial CT in a 77-year-old man with rectal carcinoma demonstrates a new tiny nodule along the posterior wall of the trachea (*arrow*). (B) Follow-up CT 6 months later demonstrates significant growth (*arrow*). Bronchoscopic resection revealed metastatic colon cancer.

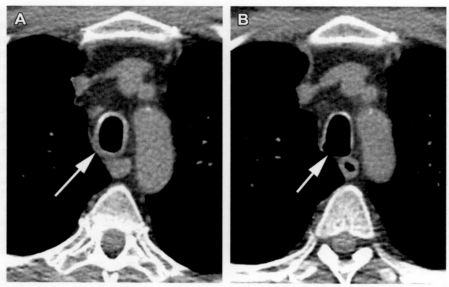

Fig. 5. (*A*) Axial CT in an immunosuppressed 44-year-old man with cough after a bone marrow transplant demonstrates subtle diffuse thickening of the tracheal wall (*arrow*). (*B*) Follow-up CT after resolution of symptoms demonstrates complete resolution of the tracheal thickening. The membranous posterior wall is now barely perceptible (*arrow*).

manifests as a dilated trachea greater than 3 cm measured 2 cm above the aortic arch.[24] MPRs are helpful in demonstrating the scalloping and outpouchings that may be seen with Mounier-Kuhn syndrome.

Paratracheal air cysts are common and usually present on the right posterior lateral wall of the trachea at the level of the thoracic inlet as an air-filled cyst that may or may not have a visible connection to the tracheal lumen. They are associated with COPD and may be seen in glassblowers.[25]

MDCT also readily demonstrates congenital abnormalities of the airways, such as tracheal bronchus, as well as the relationship of the airways to congenital abnormalities of the central vasculature.[26]

VIRTUAL ENDOSCOPY

In clinical practice, the radiologist is adept at reading scans using the axial images. However, as with MPRs, VE provides an opportunity for added information and improved display of the findings. With VE, the airway lumen is reconstructed taking advantage of the high air-to-soft tissue contrast ratio. The 3D reconstruction that results provides an endoluminal view of the trachea and is navigated using a fly-through to simulate conventional bronchoscopy. The tissue color is preset by the software package but can be modified. A threshold value of −500 HU is used to delineate between air and tracheal wall. Some

caution must be used in reconstruction, as the size of the structures depends on the reconstruction settings.[27] A trained technologist can perform the postprocessing in around 10 minutes.

Using VE involves no additional radiation. Low-dose techniques have been used in pediatric patients with foreign body aspiration with excellent or good quality in 91% of the children studied.[28] VE is usually performed during inspiration; therefore, it has a low negative predictive value for tracheomalacia, which is best demonstrated on dynamic imaging.[11]

Applications

Tracheal stenosis

VE is highly sensitive in evaluating airway obstruction when compared with the gold standard of bronchoscopy and intraoperative findings.[11] Correlation between VE and conventional bronchoscopy of stenosis contour and shape was excellent with stenosis-to-lumen ratio measures found to be within 10%.[29] One distinct advantage of VE is the ability to view beyond a high-grade obstruction that may not be passed by bronchoscopy (**Fig. 6**). In fact, some investigators suggest the combination of MDCT with MPR and VE could be considered as a substitute to direct visualization in select scenarios.[12] The use of VE reduces the overestimation of stenosis compared with axial and MPRs and correlates more closely in grading stenosis with

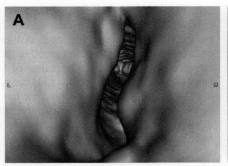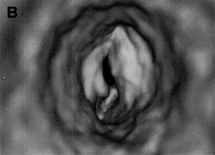

Fig. 6. Anterograde (*A*) and retrograde (*B*) VE of the postintubation stenosis seen in **Fig. 2.**

conventional bronchoscopy.[13] Compared with conventional axial MDCT, VE was slightly more accurate in evaluating significant stenosis in lung transplant. It does not replace conventional bronchoscopy but is complementary in this patient group.[30]

Airway tumors

Although VE is excellent in depiction of airway tumors, it suffers from poor sensitivity in detecting mucosal lesions.[19] VE is limited compared with visual examination in that it cannot distinguish between the color and texture of the tracheal mucosa. Of course, VE cannot sample tissue or treat lesions but has found a potential role in planning transbronchial needle aspiration of mediastinal and hilar lymph nodes.[31]

Congenital airway abnormalities

Low-dose MDCT in the pediatric population can achieve a 79% to 86% dose reduction while correctly depicting 11 of 12 airway stenoses using VE in combination with axial CT, MPRs, and SSD.[32]

Dynamic Expiratory Imaging

Dynamic imaging is useful for evaluating the trachea for narrowing during expiration. The dynamic CT protocol involves scanning the trachea at end inspiration followed by several acquisitions during dynamic expiration. The authors acquire images of the trachea typically at 8 time points during expiration (**Fig. 7**). The use of dynamic imaging is important because the trachea may be narrowest

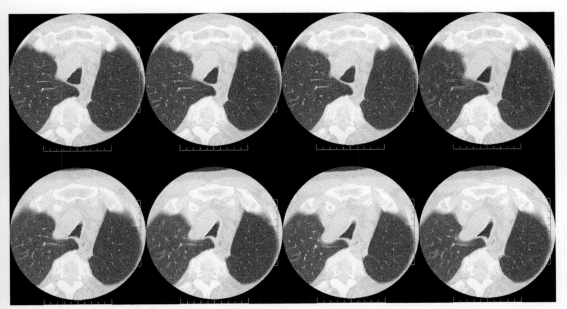

Fig. 7. Normal dynamic expiratory imaging of the trachea in a 77-year-old man demonstrates the tracheal lumen at inspiration (*top left panel*) through to expiration (*bottom right panel*).

during the process of expiration and not necessarily at end expiration.[33] Dynamic imaging could be challenging in those with hearing impairment when following breathing instructions is critical.[34] A low-dose technique may be used to limit radiation exposure from multiple acquisitions, and low-dose techniques have been validated in the literature.[35]

The inspiratory shape of the trachea will nearly always be normal in tracheomalacia.[36] Tracheomalacia is, therefore, likely underdiagnosed on routine end-inspiratory imaging. On expiratory imaging, the trachea shows a wide range of collapsibility, even in the healthy population, because of the mobile membranous posterior wall.[5] The tracheal shape on expiratory imaging is variable, but the frown configuration was seen in only 1 of 51 healthy patients and has been more commonly associated with tracheomalacia.[5,36] The degree of deformity or bowing has been classified in 4 groups as expiratory (1) through expiratory (4) depending on the degree of anterior bowing of the posterior tracheal membrane, this terminology may be applied to patients with tracheomalacia.[36,37]

The decrease in the anteroposterior and transverse diameter of the trachea on CT correlate well with the decrease in cross-sectional area.[5,37] The maximal cross-sectional area of the trachea in a set of normal patients measured in the upper trachea was 255.8 ± 61.81 mm^2. The minimal cross-sectional area of the upper trachea during expiration was 112.57 ± 49.32 mm^2, a reduction

of $54.34\% \pm 18.6$. Because a tracheal narrowing of more than 50% is commonly seen in normal patients during expiration, the study authors suggest caution when using a cutoff of 50% for the diagnosis of tracheomalacia because of the risk of overdiagnosis.[5] That being the case, dynamic expiratory CT is highly sensitive for the diagnosis of tracheomalacia, approaching that of the gold standard of bronchoscopy with only one false negative in one reported cohort (**Fig. 8**).[34]

MRI
Technical Factors and Protocol

There are many pros and cons to using MRI in imaging of the trachea. CT remains superior based on its speed and widespread availability. CT is superior in scan time, spatial resolution, and generally fewer artifacts compared with magnetic resonance (MR) examinations. MR also suffers from challenges with claustrophobia.

MRI provides superior soft tissue contrast particularly for delineating planes between the trachea and adjacent structures. In addition, MRI can visualize vasculature in the absence of intravenous contrast, which is useful when there is renal failure or an iodinated contrast allergy. MR is superior to CT in that there is no ionizing radiation.

There are limited reports of normal MR anatomy of the trachea in the literature.[38] Overall, there is limited experience in MR of the trachea, which relates to the widespread use of CT because of its speed and availability. There are select

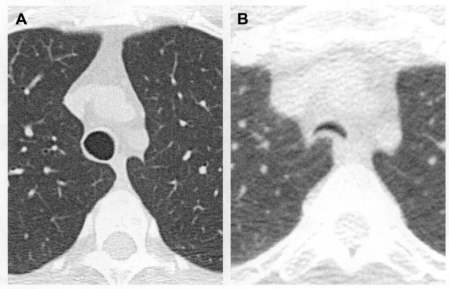

Fig. 8. (*A*) Inspiratory and (*B*) expiratory CT in a 59-year-old woman with recurrent barking cough demonstrates marked tracheal collapse consistent with tracheomalacia.

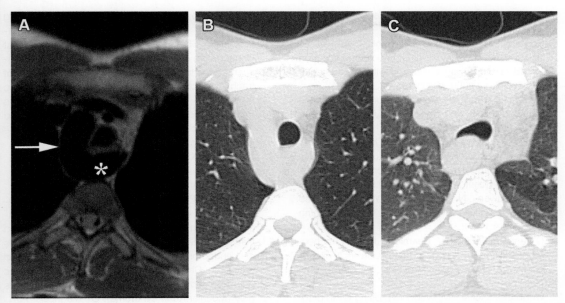

Fig. 9. (*A*) T1-weighted image in an 18-year-old man demonstrates a right-sided aortic arch (*arrow*) with aberrant left subclavian artery and diverticulum of Kommerell (*asterisk*). (*B*) Inspiratory and (*C*) expiratory axial CT demonstrates mild narrowing of the trachea during expiration.

applications whereby MR may be helpful and serve as a problem-solving tool.

Magnetic Resonance Applications

Tumors

Likely the most common indication for evaluating the trachea by MRI in adults is for assessing the extent of a mediastinal or lung tumor. The superior soft tissue contrast allows delineation of fat planes that may not be visible by CT. This delineation is important in determining the management of tracheal masses. One example of this is with endoluminal tumors whereby MR may be able to distinguish between lesions with a stalk and those with a broad base as reported in one case of a rare tracheal leiomyoma.[39]

Stenosis

MRI has been used to evaluate tracheal stenosis following percutaneous dilatational tracheostomy in 9 patients. MRI was successful in identifying scar tissue; however, the investigators did not identify any stenosis in the 9 patients, which limits the applicability of this study.[40]

Pediatric imaging

MRI is attractive in imaging pediatric patients whereby ionizing radiation is of particular concern. MR has long been used in the imaging of vascular rings in pediatric patients and can be used without the injection of intravenous contrast (**Fig. 9**).[41]

One potential application of MRI is imaging of the airways in infants using ultrashort echo times without respiratory gating when breath-hold cannot be achieved.[42]

SUMMARY

There are evolving imaging modalities available for evaluating the trachea. Each imaging modality, from MDCT, VE, dynamic expiratory imaging, and MR, provides a diverse array of applications to answer important clinical questions. Technology has advanced far beyond the plain radiography at the early stages of tracheal imaging in Dr Pearson's career to see advanced imaging play an increasingly important and complementary role to bronchoscopy in evaluating a myriad of diseases.

REFERENCES

1. Greene R, Lechner GL. "Saber-sheath" trachea: a clinical and functional study of marked coronal narrowing of the intrathoracic trachea. Radiology 1975;115(2):265–8.
2. Salour M. The steeple sign. Radiology 2000;216(2): 428–9.
3. Remy-Jardin M, Remy J, Artaud D, et al. Tracheobronchial tree: assessment with volume rendering–technical aspects. Radiology 1998;208(2):393–8.
4. Remy-Jardin M, Remy J, Artaud D, et al. Volume rendering of the tracheobronchial tree: clinical

evaluation of bronchographic images. Radiology 1998;208(3):761–70.

5. Boiselle PM, O'Donnell CR, Bankier AA, et al. Tracheal collapsibility in healthy volunteers during forced expiration: assessment with multidetector CT. Radiology 2009;252(1):255–62.

6. Gamsu G, Webb WR. Computed tomography of the trachea: normal and abnormal. AJR Am J Roentgenol 1982;139(2):321–6.

7. Hong SR, Lee YJ, Hong YJ, et al. Differentiation between mucus secretion and endoluminal tumors in the airway: analysis and comparison of CT findings. AJR Am J Roentgenol 2014;202(5):982–8.

8. Thoongsuwan N, Stern EJ. Warfarin-induced tracheobronchial calcification. J Thorac Imaging 2003;18(2):110–2.

9. O'Regan A, Fenlon HM, Beamis JF Jr, et al. Tracheobronchial amyloidosis. The Boston University experience from 1984 to 1999. Medicine (Baltimore) 2000; 79(2):69–79.

10. Webb EM, Elicker BM, Webb WR. Using CT to diagnose nonneoplastic tracheal abnormalities: appearance of the tracheal wall. AJR Am J Roentgenol 2000;174(5):1315–21.

11. Morshed K, Trojanowska A, Szymanski M, et al. Evaluation of tracheal stenosis: comparison between computed tomography virtual tracheobronchoscopy with multiplanar reformatting, flexible tracheofiberoscopy and intra-operative findings. Eur Arch Otorhinolaryngol 2011;268(4):591–7.

12. Taha MS, Mostafa BE, Fahmy M, et al. Spiral CT virtual bronchoscopy with multiplanar reformatting in the evaluation of post-intubation tracheal stenosis: comparison between endoscopic, radiological and surgical findings. Eur Arch Otorhinolaryngol 2009; 266(6):863–6.

13. Hoppe H, Walder B, Sonnenschein M, et al. Multidetector CT virtual bronchoscopy to grade tracheobronchial stenosis. AJR Am J Roentgenol 2002; 178(5):1195–200.

14. Screaton NJ, Sivasothy P, Flower CD, et al. Tracheal involvement in Wegener's granulomatosis: evaluation using spiral CT. Clin Radiol 1998;53(11):809–15.

15. Prince JS, Duhamel DR, Levin DL, et al. Nonneoplastic lesions of the tracheobronchial wall: radiologic findings with bronchoscopic correlation. Radiographics 2002;22(Spec No):S215–30.

16. Godoy MC, Saldana DA, Rao PP, et al. Multidetector CT evaluation of airway stents: what the radiologist should know. Radiographics 2014;34(7): 1793–806.

17. Righini C, Aniwidyaningsih W, Ferretti G, et al. Computed tomography measurements for airway stent insertion in malignant airway obstruction. J Bronchology Interv Pulmonol 2010;17(1):22–8.

18. Dialani V, Ernst A, Sun M, et al. MDCT detection of airway stent complications: comparison with bronchoscopy. AJR Am J Roentgenol 2008;191(5): 1576–80.

19. Finkelstein SE, Schrump DS, Nguyen DM, et al. Comparative evaluation of super high-resolution CT scan and virtual bronchoscopy for the detection of tracheobronchial malignancies. Chest 2003;124(5): 1834–40.

20. Park CM, Goo JM, Lee HJ, et al. Tumors in the tracheobronchial tree: CT and FDG PET features. Radiographics 2009;29(1):55–71.

21. Kim Y, Lee KS, Yoon JH, et al. Tuberculosis of the trachea and main bronchi: CT findings in 17 patients. AJR Am J Roentgenol 1997;168(4):1051–6.

22. Logan PM, Primack SL, Miller RR, et al. Invasive aspergillosis of the airways: radiographic, CT, and pathologic findings. Radiology 1994;193(2):383–8.

23. Nathan SD, Shorr AF, Schmidt ME, et al. Aspergillus and endobronchial abnormalities in lung transplant recipients. Chest 2000;118(2):403–7.

24. Shin MS, Jackson RM, Ho KJ. Tracheobronchomegaly (Mounier-Kuhn syndrome): CT diagnosis. AJR Am J Roentgenol 1988;150(4):777–9.

25. Goo JM, Im JG, Ahn JM, et al. Right paratracheal air cysts in the thoracic inlet: clinical and radiologic significance. AJR Am J Roentgenol 1999;173(1):65–70.

26. Chassagnon G, Morel B, Carpentier E, et al. Tracheobronchial branching abnormalities: lobe-based classification scheme. Radiographics 2016; 36(2):358–73.

27. Summers RM, Shaw DJ, Shelhamer JH. CT virtual bronchoscopy of simulated endobronchial lesions: effect of scanning, reconstruction, and display settings and potential pitfalls. AJR Am J Roentgenol 1998;170(4):947–50.

28. Kosucu P, Ahmetoglu A, Koramaz I, et al. Low-dose MDCT and virtual bronchoscopy in pediatric patients with foreign body aspiration. AJR Am J Roentgenol 2004;183(6):1771–7.

29. Burke AJ, Vining DJ, McGuirt WF Jr, et al. Evaluation of airway obstruction using virtual endoscopy. Laryngoscope 2000;110(1):23–9.

30. McAdams HP, Palmer SM, Erasmus JJ, et al. Bronchial anastomotic complications in lung transplant recipients: virtual bronchoscopy for noninvasive assessment. Radiology 1998;209(3):689–95.

31. McAdams HP, Goodman PC, Kussin P. Virtual bronchoscopy for directing transbronchial needle aspiration of hilar and mediastinal lymph nodes: a pilot study. AJR Am J Roentgenol 1998;170(5):1361–4.

32. Honnef D, Wildberger JE, Das M, et al. Value of virtual tracheobronchoscopy and bronchography from 16-slice multidetector-row spiral computed tomography for assessment of suspected tracheobronchial stenosis in children. Eur Radiol 2006;16(8):1684–91.

33. Baroni RH, Feller-Kopman D, Nishino M, et al. Tracheobronchomalacia: comparison between end-expiratory and dynamic expiratory CT for evaluation

of central airway collapse. Radiology 2005;235(2): 635–41.

34. Lee KS, Sun MR, Ernst A, et al. Comparison of dynamic expiratory CT with bronchoscopy for diagnosing airway malacia: a pilot evaluation. Chest 2007;131(3):758–64.

35. Zhang J, Hasegawa I, Feller-Kopman D, et al. 2003 AUR Memorial Award. Dynamic expiratory volumetric CT imaging of the central airways: comparison of standard-dose and low-dose techniques. Acad Radiol 2003;10(7):719–24.

36. Boiselle PM, Ernst A. Tracheal morphology in patients with tracheomalacia: prevalence of inspiratory lunate and expiratory "frown" shapes. J Thorac Imaging 2006;21(3):190–6.

37. Stern EJ, Graham CM, Webb WR, et al. Normal trachea during forced expiration: dynamic CT measurements. Radiology 1993;187(1):27–31.

38. Reed JM, O'Connor DM, Myer CM 3rd. Magnetic resonance imaging determination of tracheal orientation in normal children. Practical implications. Arch Otolaryngol Head Neck Surg 1996;122(6): 605–8.

39. Maehara M, Ikeda K, Ohmura N, et al. Leiomyoma of the trachea: CT and MRI findings. Radiat Med 2006; 24(9):643–5.

40. Callanan V, Gillmore K, Field S, et al. The use of magnetic resonance imaging to assess tracheal stenosis following percutaneous dilatational tracheostomy. J Laryngol Otol 1997;111(10):953–7.

41. Bisset GS 3rd, Strife JL, Kirks DR, et al. Vascular rings: MR imaging. AJR Am J Roentgenol 1987; 149(2):251–6.

42. Niwa T, Nozawa K, Aida N. Visualization of the airway in infants with MRI using pointwise encoding time reduction with radial acquisition (PETRA). J Magn Reson Imaging 2017;45(3):839–44.

Surgical Disorders of the Airway

Tracheal Injuries Complicating Prolonged Intubation and Tracheostomy

Joel D. Cooper, MD

KEYWORDS

- Postintubation airway complications • Tracheal stenosis • Prolonged intubation

KEY POINTS

- Airway complications following prolonged ventilator assistance remains a significant but largely preventable problem.
- Postintubation tracheal stenosis most commonly results from overinflation of the cuff causing pressure necrosis of the adjacent tracheal wall.
- Symptoms, including increasing shortness of breath and wheezing, usually present between 4 and 8 weeks after extubation and are frequently misdiagnosed as asthma.
- Malpositioning of an endotracheal tube cuff in the subglottic region may result in subsequent stenosis at that level, following as little as 2 days of exposure.
- A high tracheostomy site, at the level of the cricoid cartilage or the first tracheal ring, may result in partial or complete subglottic stricture and the inability to safely decannulate the tracheostomy tube.

INTRODUCTION

Injuries to the upper airway related to the use of endotracheal and tracheostomy tubes for ventilatory assistance reflect a common theme: innovative advances in the medical field often generate a new set of complications, which then generate further advances designed to reduce or eliminate such consequences. During the authors' preparation of this article, written in tribute to Dr F.G. Pearson, there were many long pauses for reflection on the remarkable advances in cardiothoracic surgery, anesthetic management, and postoperative care that have occurred since the author was a surgical intern in 1964.

HISTORY OF POSITIVE-PRESSURE VENTILATION

The oldest recorded surgical procedure on the airway is in the Edwin Smith Papyrus, an ancient Egyptian medical text thought to date around 1600 BCE. It illustrates what is thought to be a tracheotomy to provide an emergency airway. The use of tracheotomy, with or without insertion of a tracheostomy tube, was used almost exclusively for treatment of upper airway obstruction until the latter half of the nineteenth century. Several articles have chronicled the history and evolution of tracheostomy use.[1–3]

The development of thoracic surgery, the ability to safely operate within the chest, posed a unique problem. Specifically, opening the chest and exposing the lung to atmospheric pressure eliminated the normal negative differential pressure between the pleural space and the upper airway, allowing the lung to collapse from its unopposed elastic recoil. Endotracheal intubation was used by Vesalius in 1543 for artificial respiration. In 1895, Tuffier modified an endotracheal tube by adding an inflatable cuff around it to allow positive

Disclosure: The author has nothing to disclose.

Department of Surgery, Division of Thoracic Surgery, Hospital of the University of Pennsylvania, University of Pennsylvania, 3400 Spruce Street, White 6, Philadelphia, PA 19104, USA

E-mail address: joel.cooper@uphs.upenn.edu

thoracic.theclinics.com

pressure to be applied to the lung. Nonetheless, for some reason, this technique was not used in the early days of thoracic surgery. Desiring to operate on patients with esophageal malignancies, von Mikulicz charged his disciple Sauerbruch with the task of solving the problem. Sauerbruch's solution was a negative pressure operating room chamber, in which the operating theater was a sealed room in which the pressure could be reduced by 10 to 20 cm below atmospheric pressure. The patient's head went through a hole in the wall with the neck surrounded by a sealing cuff so that the mouth and nose were exposed to atmospheric pressure on one side of the wall while the chest (and the operating staff) was exposed to a negative differential pressure on the operating room side. Thus, when the chest was open, the lung could remain inflated because subatmospheric pressure was maintained in the chamber and anesthesia was administered by the anesthetist outside the chamber. By the summer of 1904, von Mikulicz had performed 16 pulmonary or esophageal cases on patients using this technique.

Meltzer and Auer, in New York in 1909, recognized the advantage of using positive intraoperative pressure with an endotracheal tube but the reputation of Sauerbruch and von Mikulicz, and their continued advocacy of the negative pressure chamber, suppressed the acceptance of positive-pressure ventilation with an endotracheal tube for almost a decade.

Until the 1950s, positive-pressure ventilation was reserved almost exclusively for intraoperative anesthetic management using a facial mask, uncuffed endotracheal tubes with pharyngeal packing to prevent air-leakage, or cuffed endotracheal tubes. The extension of positive-pressure ventilation to the treatment of respiratory failure resulted from the poliomyelitis epidemic in Copenhagen in 1952 as a substitute for the use of the iron lung. Its routine use for postoperative respiratory support occurred a decade later, primarily in association with the development of cardiac surgery. Until that time, there were no postoperative intensive care units and the concept of electively providing postoperative respiratory support was not generally adopted. This is sadly illustrated by the authors' reminiscence, as an intern in 1964, of a woman in her late 20s with myasthenia gravis who had undergone median sternotomy for excision of a thymoma. Postoperatively, the patient was in respiratory distress for several days with labored breathing and secretion retention. It was uncertain whether or not the problem was a myasthenic crisis mandating higher doses of steroids and anticholinesterase medications, or a cholinergic crisis due to excessive administration of anticholinesterase agents. At the time, the notion of intubating and ventilating the patient was apparently not considered and the patient succumbed.

ETIOLOGIC FACTORS OF POSTINTUBATION UPPER AIRWAY INJURY

With the advent and proliferation of subspecialty intensive care units, which included the provision of mechanical respiratory support, the use of tracheostomy markedly increased and, not surprisingly, complications of this procedure were not uncommon. By and large, these were early postoperative complications, including wound hemorrhage, or displacement or secretion obstruction of the tube. Increasing experience eliminated most of these early complications but, as patients began to survive longer periods of respiratory assistance, a new group of late complications from the use of cuffed endotracheal tubes or tracheostomy tubes developed. There were reports documenting an increased incidence of postintubation tracheal stenosis as high as 20%. Strictures were reported both in the region of the tracheostomy stoma and at the level of the inflatable cuff.

In 1968, Pearson and colleagues reported on 24 individuals with postintubation tracheal strictures, over two-thirds of which were thought to arise at the level of the stoma.[4] Over a similar period, Grillo[5] reported surgical management in 31 postintubation strictures, 27 of which were thought to be at the cuff site and 4 at the stomal site.

TRACHEAL STENOSIS AT THE CUFF SITE

In 1965, the author, under the direction of Dr Grillo, performed autopsy examination of the larynx and trachea on 30 patients who died in the hospital while receiving respiratory assistance through cuffed endotracheal or tracheostomy tubes.[6] The duration of intubation before death ranged from 1 day to 8 weeks. The gross and microscopic evaluation revealed a consistent pattern of damage to the tracheal wall correlating with the site of the balloon cuff. In general, the longer the duration of mechanical ventilation the greater the injury to the trachea. Early changes included mucosal hemorrhage and ulceration, which progressed to deeper ulcerations exposing portions of the cartilaginous rings. With longer exposure, these ulcerations increased in extent, resulting in fragmentation and dissolution of adjacent cartilaginous rings. This left a segment of trachea without support and full-thickness damage to the tracheal wall. It was concluded that in survivors this segment progressed to cicatricial fibrosis and contraction, resulting in tracheal stenosis (**Fig. 1**).

The same pattern of tracheal injury at the cuff site was described in a prospective study by Pearson and colleagues.[7] They performed postdecannulation bronchoscopic observations on subjects who had received respiratory assistance with a cuffed tracheostomy tube. Every subject exhibited significant damage, primarily at the site of the cuff. This finding was essentially the same whether a cuffed tracheostomy tube or endotracheal tube had been utilized.

Further studies confirmed that tracheal injury at the cuff site was primarily due to pressure necrosis caused by the nature of the very elastic, distensible cuffs used at the time on tracheostomy tubes and endotracheal tubes.[8] These elastic cuffs, when opened to the air, would shrink tightly against the outer wall of the tube for ease of insertion. However, they required considerable pressure for inflation (between 180 and 250 mm Hg), rendering them relatively rigid and noncompliant. They created a seal between the tube and the airway by deforming the contours of the trachea to match the eccentric rigid contours of the cuff. The high-volume low-pressure cuffs that were subsequently developed required only enough inflation pressure to match the pressure in the airway and easily adapted their shape to the contours of the trachea, creating very little resulting pressure on the tracheal wall.[9] With the advent of these cuffs, the incidence of postintubation tracheal stenosis at the site of the cuffs has markedly diminished. However, even a high-volume low-pressure cuff can cause pressure necrosis of the trachea if it is unnecessarily overinflated.

STOMAL STENOSIS

A less common cause of postintubation tracheal stenosis occurs at the site of the tracheostomy stoma whereby loss of the anterior supporting portion of the cartilaginous arch is lost either due to too large a tracheostomy stoma or by enlargement of the stomal site by leverage on the tracheostomy tube, often due to its unsupported attachment to the ventilator tubing. Following extubation, the resulting defect in the anterior portion of the trachea may cause inward collapse of the lateral walls, creating a so-called A-frame stenosis. On bronchoscopy this appears more distal, very much like a second set of vocal cords in the upper trachea with an acute angle anteriorly between the lateral walls of the tracheal segment, which diverge as they angle posteriorly to join the membranous wall (**Fig. 2**). The tracheal mucosa and underlying cartilaginous rings of the lateral walls look essentially normal, as does the membranous wall. Thus, the anterior-posterior diameter of the stenotic segment may be fairly normal, whereas the lateral diameter is compromised by the collapse of the lateral walls. Early on, the lateral walls are not fused to each other anteriorly and the lateral dimensions of the airway can increase and decrease with the respiratory cycle, causing little resistance to airflow with routine activities.

Another potential complication at the tracheostomy site may result from the buildup of granulation tissue in the airway, usually along the superior border of the stoma. This can usually be managed with 1 or 2 endoscopic debridements, cauterization, steroid injections, or short-term stenting with a silicone T-tube.

POSTINTUBATION SUBGLOTTIC STENOSIS

The spectrum of postintubation injuries has shifted somewhat in recent years. Formerly, postintubation stenosis either at the cuff site or at the stomal site occurred in the upper half of the trachea somewhere between the second ring and the midpoint of the trachea. However, postintubation stenosis at or just below the cricoid cartilage has become increasingly common and presents a more challenging technical

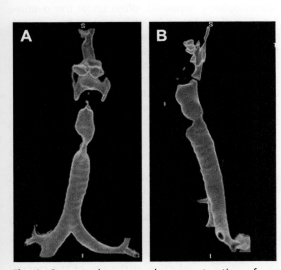

Fig. 1. Computed tomography reconstruction of upper airway in patient with posttracheostomy stenosis at the cuff site. The circumferential scarring and progressive airway narrowing typically presents 4 to 8 weeks after extubation with increasing dyspnea on exertion, wheezing, and stridor. (*A*) Posteroanterior. (*B*) Lateral.

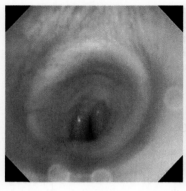 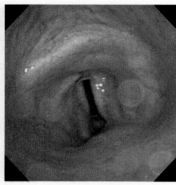

Fig. 2. Two cases of posttracheostomy stricture at the stomal site due to loss of anterior support involving 1 or more tracheal rings. The side walls have collapsed but the anterior-posterior diameter of the airway is usually maintained. The lateral walls often remain mobile. Clinical presentation in the form of dyspnea may not occur for years or even decades when scarring or ossification of the anterior hinge results in a fixed, slit-like narrowing.

problem as far as resection is concerned. Such injuries are usually caused by high placement of a tracheostomy tube with consequent injury and infection at the level of the cricoid cartilage. The resultant damage may extend proximally to within 1 cm of the vocal cords. Such damage may lead to complete obliteration of the airway in the subglottic region, leaving the patient dependent on a tracheostomy tube and unable to speak (**Fig. 3**). The reason for this increasing number of high airway strictures is uncertain but the use of percutaneous tracheostomies with malpositioning of the tracheostomy site may play a role. Furthermore, emergency placement of a tracheostomy tube in patients who are now more likely to survive complex trauma, and the rising incidence of morbid obesity making even elective tracheostomy difficult to site at a desirable position, may contribute.

A second, and more preventable, cause of post-intubation subglottic stricture is the malpositioning of an endotracheal tube such that the cuff is located at the level of the cricoid cartilage, which is the most narrow, rigid, and nondistensible part of the airway. At this site, even modest overinflation of the cuff can cause severe airway injury and result in subsequent stenosis after as few as 2 days of exposure of the airway to the overinflated cuff. The usual scenario is urgent or emergent endotracheal intubation in the field or in the emergency ward following acute traumatic or medical emergency. The priority in this situation is to quickly establish an airway and transfer the patient to the hospital, the radiology unit, or the operating room. The tube is inserted as quickly as possible, often under difficult circumstances, and then the cuff is rapidly inflated using the so-called push and run technique; that is, inflating the cuff with a syringe until it feels firm, confirming the ability to ventilate, and rapidly transporting the patient. Subsequent chest radiographs, when retrospectively reviewed, often show the overinflated cuff in the subglottic region for several days before it is removed, changed, or repositioned. As noted, the result of this injury may be subsequent complete obliteration of the subglottic airway (**Fig. 4**). This complication, like that resulting from a high tracheostomy site, is significantly more complex to deal with than is a segmental stricture in the upper trachea.

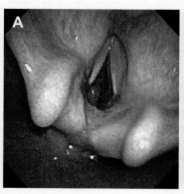 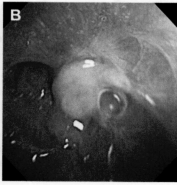

Fig. 3. (*A*) Subglottic stricture at level of cricoid cartilage in 18-year-old man who sustained a gunshot to the mandible. Emergency intubation was followed by elective tracheostomy at the time of the mandibular repair. (*B*) Injury and infection at the site of the stoma, adjacent to the cricoid arch, resulted in subsequent complete obliteration of the airway. Successful laryngotracheal resection was accomplished at a later date.

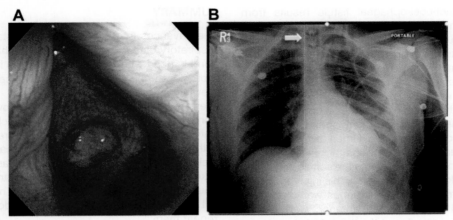

Fig. 4. (*A*) Subglottic stenosis with complete airway obliteration at the level of the cricoid arch in a 23-year-old man secondary to endotracheal intubation following spontaneous subarachnoid hemorrhage. (*B*) Retrospective review of postadmission chest radiographs revealed that the site of the endotracheal tube cuff (see *arrow*)was in the subglottic region for 2 to 3 days before the tube was removed. Symptoms of critical upper airway narrowing occurred 2 months later, requiring emergency tracheostomy. Successful laryngotracheal resection was performed at a later date.

CLINICAL PRESENTATION OF POSTINTUBATION TRACHEAL STENOSIS

The presenting symptoms of patients who develop postintubation upper airway obstruction vary greatly depending on the nature of the airway injury. If the stenosis is within 2 to 3 cm of the vocal cords, caused either by traumatic intubation or injury to the cricotracheal junction from an endotracheal tube cuff or a highly placed tracheostomy stoma, airway obstruction may first be recognized in hospital by the inability to safely decannulate a tracheostomy tube due to an inadequate airway proximal to the tracheostomy stoma. More often, however, postintubation cuff stenosis presents as increasing shortness of breath beginning 4 to 8 weeks after decannulation because progressive scarring and contraction of the airway occurs at the site of a cuff injury. These patients experience increasing exertional dyspnea and wheezing, which is frequently misdiagnosed as asthma. Only when the stenosis reaches a critical stage is the true nature of the problem recognized.

Unlike the stenosis resulting from a cuff injury that is circumferential, rigid, and fixed, narrowing at the stomal site may be pliable and offer little or no resistance even to passage of a rigid bronchoscope. However, over time the tracheal narrowing may become fixed and, for this reason, the presentation of stomal stenosis is often more subtle, less progressive, and may not create a significant functional problem until years or even decades later. Presumably this is due to ossification and fixation of the anterior hinge joining the lateral tracheal walls and resulting in a fixed stenosis. The author recently encountered such a case in which significant symptoms resulting from a stomal stenosis first occurred more than 65 years after the patient had undergone temporary tracheostomy at age 5 for an episode of epiglottitis.

LARYNGEAL INJURY

Formerly, injury to the larynx at the glottic level from an endotracheal tube used for prolonged ventilatory support was not uncommon. This included ulceration of the arytenoid cartilages, dislocation of an arytenoid cartilage, or interarytenoid scarring and stricture. Such injuries are particularly prone to occur if an oversized endotracheal tube is used or is left in position for longer than a week, especially in a patient who is semiconscious or unconscious and thrashing around in the bed, causing repeated trauma between the tube and the larynx. Improved design of endotracheal tubes and devices to provide stable fixation of the tube to the patient's head almost completely eliminated this problem. In patients who are alert and cooperative, or are being paralyzed, and with proper fixation of the endotracheal tube, and routine alternating of its position from side to side, endotracheal tube intubation can be safely maintained for 1 to 2 weeks without injury and without the need to convert to tracheostomy.

OTHER POSTINTUBATION INJURIES

In addition to tracheal stricture, 2 other serious consequences of tracheostomy tubes are tracheoinnominate artery fistula and tracheoesophageal fistula. Tracheoesophageal fistula results from pressure necrosis of the membranous wall of the trachea due to an overinflated or high-pressure cuff causing erosion through the membranous wall and into the lumen of the adjacent esophagus. This process occurs over a period of time such that the membranous wall of the trachea initially fuses to the outer wall of the esophagus. As a result, when the subsequent communication is established between the lumen of the trachea and the lumen of the esophagus, there is no air leakage from the trachea into the soft tissue planes of the neck. This distinguishes this injury from surgical trauma to the membranous wall of the trachea and the adjacent anterior wall of the esophagus occurring at the time of tracheostomy, in which case subcutaneous air is radiologically obvious in the neck.

Tracheoinnominate artery fistula is an uncommon but frequently fatal late consequence of tracheostomy. This communication between the anterior wall of the trachea and posterior wall of the innominate artery may occur in a similar fashion as tracheoesophageal fistula, namely pressure necrosis through the anterior wall of the trachea at the cuff site. However, in the author's experience, it has more commonly been associated with erosion by the anterior wall of the elbow of the tracheostomy tube into the superior-posterior wall of the innominate artery. This may be due to a tracheostomy stoma fashioned too distally or, more likely, from gradual enlargement of the tracheostomy stoma inferiorly due to downward tugging on the tracheostomy tube by the attached ventilator tubing. In addition, a purulent tracheostomy wound due to contamination from the airway and/or inadequate wound care may contribute. The premonitory hemorrhage that usually occurs before terminal exsanguination presents as bleeding out of the neck wound or out the nasopharynx rather than through the tracheostomy tube because the innominate artery fenestration is proximal to the tracheostomy cuff which may protect the distal airway. If bleeding first presents through the tracheostomy tube rather than around it, the source of bleeding may be pulmonary hemorrhage and not tracheoinnominate artery fistula.

For an outstanding, well-organized, systematic, and highly referenced article on postintubation injuries, the reader is referred to the 1971 review by Harley.[10]

SUMMARY

The advances made in ventilator assistance and respiratory care over the last 50 years have gone hand in hand with remarkable progress in cardiothoracic surgery and other surgical specialties. Inevitably, the widespread use of positive-pressure ventilation has generated its own set of complications, as described in this article. Fortunately, such complications are usually preventable if the factors resulting in such complications are well understood and if appropriate measures are taken to prevent them. Nowhere is Santayana's cautionary aphorism more relevant, "Those who fail to learn the lessons of history are doomed to repeat them."

REFERENCES

1. Goodall EW. The story of tracheostomy. Br J Childs Dis 1934;31:167–76, 253.72.

2. Frost EA. Tracing the tracheostomy. Ann Otol Rhinol Laryngol 1976;85(5 Pt. 1):618–24.

3. Eavey RD. The evolution of tracheostomy. In: Myers EN, Stool SE, Johnson JT, editors. Tracheostomy. New York: Churchill Livingstone; 1985. p. 1–11.

4. Pearson FG, Goldberg M, da Silva AJ. A prospective study of tracheal injury complicating tracheostomy with a cuffed tube. Ann Otol Rhinol Laryngol 1968;77:867.

5. Grillo HC. The management of tracheal stenosis following assisted respiration. J Thorac Cardiovasc Surg 1969;57:52–71.

6. Cooper JD, Grillo HC. The evolution of tracheal injury due to ventilator assistance through cuffed tubes. A pathologic study. Ann Surg 1969;169:334.

7. Pearson FG, Goldberg M, da Silva AJ. Tracheal stenosis complicating tracheostomy with cuffed tubes. Clinical experience and observations from a prospective study. Arch Surg 1968;97:380.

8. Cooper JD, Grillo HC. Experimental production and prevention of injury due to cuffed tracheal tubes. Surg Gynecol Obstet 1969;129:1235.

9. Grillo HC, Cooper JD, Geffin B, et al. A low pressure cuff for tracheostomy tubes to minimize tracheal injury: a comparative clinical trial. J Thorac Cardiovasc Surg 1971;62:898.

10. Harley HRS. Laryngotracheal obstruction complicating tracheostomy or endotracheal intubation with assisted respiration. Thorax 1971;26:493–533.

Biology of Adenoid Cystic Carcinoma of the Tracheobronchial Tree and Principles of Management

Donna E. Maziak, MDCM, MSc, FRCSC, FACS

KEYWORDS

- Adenoid cystic carcinoma • Tracheal tumors • Surgical resection

KEY POINTS

- Adenoid cystic carcinoma of the trachea is a rare tumor.
- The mainstay of treatment remains surgical resection, even in the presence of positive margins or metastatic disease.
- Long-term follow-up is required with patients presenting late and surviving with recurrent disease for years.

BIOLOGY OF ADENOID CYSTIC CARCINOMA

Adenoid cystic carcinoma (ACC) of the airway is an uncommon malignant tumor, of salivary gland-type. It is the second most common primary malignant tracheal neoplasm after squamous cell carcinoma. Histologically, it originates from the submucosal glands and is composed of small round cells arranged in a cribriform manner, with larger paler cells forming clumps and pseudoacini. The clinical and pathologic features of ACC of the trachea were first reported in 1859 by Billroth.[1] It was previously referred to as a benign glandular neoplasm or adenoma but is now considered a low-grade bronchial carcinoma that is malignant, frequently locally invasive, and often late to metastasize.

Patients typically are middle-aged, with an equal preponderance of men and women. There are no studies that have found an association with smoking or excessive alcohol consumption. It is most often slow-growing and diagnosis is often delayed for 5 or more years. Symptoms vary according to location of the tumor in the airway. This tumor tends to be locally infiltrative between the tracheal rings, producing the so-called iceberg effect, with late metastasis. These tumors will bulge into the lumen and cause symptoms of tracheal obstruction and even hemoptysis. Patients most commonly present with dyspnea but may also have wheezing, cough, hemoptysis, and stridor. Often, early in the presentation, patients are misdiagnosed with asthma or bronchitis, and are mistreated.

In recent years, advances have been made in genetic mutation studies, such as microarray, fluorescent in situ hybridization, and microsatellite polymerase chain reaction. All have been performed in ACC for better understanding of its pathogenesis and potential biomarkers that may affect treatment and prognosis. Thus far, high levels of *ki-67* and p63 have strongly correlated with a decreased survival rate. Terminal deoxynucleotidyl transferase mediated dUTP nick end labelling (TUNEL), an assay for apoptosis rates (if high levels of staining), has correlated with increased incidence

Disclosure: The author has nothing to disclose.
Surgical Oncology, Division of Thoracic Surgery, Ottawa Hospital–General Division, University of Ottawa, 501 Smyth Road 6NW-6364, Ottawa, Ontario K1H 8L6, Canada
E-mail address: dmaziak@ottawahospital.on.ca

Thorac Surg Clin 28 (2018) 145–148
https://doi.org/10.1016/j.thorsurg.2018.01.002

of metastasis, extracapsular spread, grade, and stage; thereby decreasing survival rates.[2] Some tumors have displayed a fused gene product of chromosomes 6 and 9, MYB-FIB gene, and this may hold the key transformation of normal healthy cells into ACC. Individuals with KIT expression, a mast cell growth factor receptor, have shown response to imatinib, a targeted chemotherapy.

PATHOLOGIC FEATURES OF ADENOID CYSTIC CARCINOMA

The tumor resembles those arising in the salivary glands. Its growth may be polypoid and sometimes annular, causing luminal obstruction. It is usually nonencapsulated, characteristically growing within the submucosal layer, thereby often appearing for some distance from the mucosal abnormality, which is often only the tip of the iceberg. Perineural and lymphatic spread is common. It is thought that the traditional tumor-node-metastasis (TNM) staging for malignancy cannot be applied to ACC because of its unique pathologic features.

There is a correlation between 3 histologic subtypes of these tumors and prognosis[3]:

1. Cribriform, the most common, has prominent pseudocysts surrounded by uniform basaloid cells with few cytoplasm and is arranged in well-defined nests of variable sizes. These have the best prognosis (**Figs. 1** and **2**).
2. Trabecular has basaloid cells arranged in nests surrounded by variable amounts of eosinophilic hyalinized stroma (**Fig. 3**).
3. Solid type has basaloid cells that aggregate without tubular or cystic formation; the tumor cells are larger with mitotic figures and comedonecrosis (**Fig. 4**). These have the poorest prognosis.

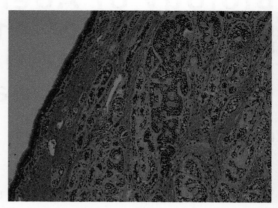

Fig. 2. ACC cribriform pattern subbronchial mucosa H&E original magnification × 1.

Usually, these patterns are mixed and pure patterns are very rare. The percentage of each pattern forms the basis of the grading system created in 1984 based on ACC in salivary glands.[4] From grades 1 to 3, there is a decreasing percentage of cribriform or tubular pattern (grade 1 has no solid component, grade 2 has <30% solid component) with an increasing percentage of solid component (grade 3 has >30% solid component).

Hematoxylin-eosin stain remains the gold standard by which the diagnosis is made; however, confusion with carcinoid or mucinous adenocarcinoma can occur. Further immunostaining may be required, including wide spectrum keratin, CK 7, actin, p63 and brain-derived neurotrophic factor.

PRINCIPLES OF MANAGEMENT

Diagnostic tissue biopsy by bronchoscopy and evaluation by an experienced pathologist is required given the orphan nature of this tumor. Further evaluation is required with computed

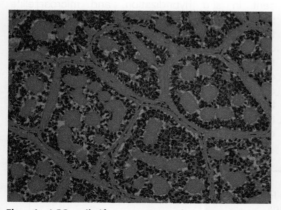

Fig. 1. ACC cribriform pattern hematoxylin-eosin (H&E) original magnification × 1 with islands and nests, with luminal matrix.

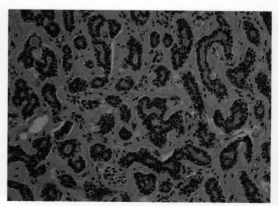

Fig. 3. ACC tubular pattern H&E original magnification × 1, with gland-like spaces.

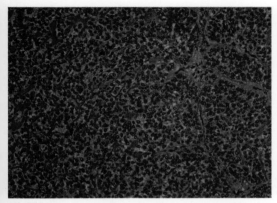

Fig. 4. ACC solid pattern H&E original magnification × 1, insular, with scant matrix.

tomography (CT) scan, bronchoscopy, and PET-CT scan. CT scans with 3 dimensional reconstruction and bronchoscopy help assess the extent of the disease and plan for surgical resection. PET-CT scans are more helpful in detecting recurrences or metastasis. Dr FG Pearson always stood by the mantra that "if you plan to operate, you have to do the bronchoscopy yourself!" Further investigations require a pulmonary function test, which is expected to show an obstructive pattern and flattening of the flow volume loop. Because lymph node status does not tend to influence survival, cervical mediastinoscopy or endobronchial ultrasound are not routinely used in the preoperative assessment.

The mainstay of treatment remains surgical resection. There is a role for postoperative adjuvant radiation for positive resection margin. Radiation for lymphatic involvement is controversial. Because ACC is characterized by indolent but progressive local growth with perineural and lymphatic invasion, resection provides excellent palliation even in the presence of metastatic disease. Patients can survive another 10 or more years, even if they presented initially with metastases.

The most frequent site of occurrence of tracheal ACC is in the distal third of the trachea. The principles of tracheal resection and primary reconstruction have been described excellently in Douglas Mathisen's article, "Distal Tracheal Resection and Reconstruction: State of the Art and Lessons Learned," in this issue. Of course, resection will often entail carinal resection and, at times, is accompanied with lobectomy. In the early years of resection, Marlex mesh grafts were entertained to help increase the length of trachea that could be resected but there is no longer need for its use in reconstruction. The advancement of surgical techniques, anesthesia, and better knowledge of the anatomy and releasing procedures has allowed almost half of the trachea to be resected and still obtain a primary anastomosis. Better understanding of the biology of the disease supported the idea of grossly negative margins, accepting microscopically positive margins secondarily to submucosal and perineural involvement.

Airway and radial margins are important prognostic indicators for long-term survival; invasion of adjacent organs have not seemed to affect survival. Studies showed no correlation between survival and lymph node status. However, perineural growth has shown a trend to decrease survival. In **Table 1**, various series (although not randomized controlled trials) showed comparable 5-year survival rates of 52% to 79% and 10-year survival of 29% to 56%.[5–9] Surgical

Table 1
Reported results of resection for adenoid cystic carcinoma of the airway

	Grillo & Mathisen,[5,6] 1990	Perelman,[7] 1987	Regnard et al,[8] 1996	Pearson,[9] 1996
Year of Publication	1990/2004	1980	1996	1996
Number of Subjects	60/133	56	65	38
Years of Follow-up	26/40	20	23	32
Operative mortality	8 (13%)/14 (7.3%)	8 (14%)	—	3 (9%)
Actuarial Survival (%)				
5 y	—/52	66	73	79
10 y	—/29	56	57	51
Mean Survival (mo)				
Radiation only	39/—	—	—	74
Resection and Radiation	108/—	—	—	88

resection seemed to offer the best survival compared with radiation alone. The results of adjuvant radiation continue to be controversial. Some studies showed a higher survival rate in subjects with complete resection and negative margins compared with incomplete resection or unresectable tumors; however, others showed no difference. There was no correlation between lymph node status and survival.

Long-term follow-up is essential in patients with ACC of the airway. Local recurrence can occur as late as 27 years but most are within 10 years. Even with metastatic disease, most commonly to the lung, most occurred later than 8 years, and most patients lived another 3 to 7 years after the diagnosis.

SUMMARY

I remember the premise under which Dr FG Pearson and I decided to write up his experience with primary ACC the airway.[9] I was the chief resident on the service at the time and, in preparation for a carinal resection for ACC, there were precious few publications to read on the topic. You would never go to the operating room unprepared. Dr Pearson always said the best residents were the ones he learned something from. As the chief resident, you never wanted to disappoint Dr Pearson. On completion of the case that day, we commenced the review of his experience of ACC at the Toronto General Hospital.

REFERENCES

1. Billroth T. Beobachtungen über geschwülsteder Speicheldrüsen. Virchous Arch Pathol Anat 1859;17: 357–75.
2. Liu J, Chunbo S, Tan ML, et al. The molecular biology of adenoid cystic carcinoma. Head Neck 2012; 34(11):1665–77.
3. Jaso J, Malhotra R. Adenoid cystic carcinoma. Arch Pathol Lab Med 2011;135:511–5.
4. Szanto PA, Luna MA, Tortoledo ME, et al. Histologic grading of adenoid cystic carcinoma of the salivary glands. Cancer 1984;54(6):1062–9.
5. Grillo HC, Mathisen DJ. Primary tracheal tumors: treatment and results. Ann Thorac Surg 1990;49: 67–77.
6. Gaissert HA, Grillo HC, Shadmehr MB, et al. Long-term survival after resection of primary adenoid cystic and squamous cell carcinoma of the trachea and carinal. Ann Thorac Surg 2004;78:1889–97.
7. Perelman MI, Koroleva N. Surgery of the tracheal. In: Grillo HC, Eschapasse H, editors. International trends in general thoracic surgery: major challenges, vol. 2. Philadelphia: WB Saunders; 1987. p. 91–110.
8. Regnard JF, Fourquier P, Lavasseur P, et al. Results and prognostic factors in resections of primary tracheal tumours: a multicenter retrospective study. J Thorac Cardiovasc Surg 1996;111:808–14.
9. Maziak DE, Todd TRJ, Keshavjee SH, et al. Adenoid cystic carcinoma of the airway: thirty-two year experience. J Thorac Cardiovasc Surg 1996;112:1522–32.

Pathology of Primary Tracheobronchial Malignancies Other than Adenoid Cystic Carcinomas

Darroch Moores, MD, FRCSC[a],*, Paresh Mane, MD, MCh[b]

KEYWORDS

- Tracheal tumors • Pathology • Adenoid cystic carcinoma • Squamous cell carcinoma
- Mucoepidermoid carcinoma

KEY POINTS

- Most primary tracheal tumors are malignant.
- Malignancy of larynx and bronchi are much more likely than trachea.
- Tracheal tumors are most likely due to direct extension for surrounding tumors.
- Squamous cell carcinoma and adenoid cystic carcinoma make up about two-thirds of adult primary tracheal tumors.
- Because of their predominantly local growth pattern, malignant salivary gland–type tumors show a better outcome than other histologic types.

INTRODUCTION

Primary tracheal tumors (PTT) are relatively rare; their diagnosis is often late because the symptoms are noncharacteristic, and the signs only appear when more than 60% of the lumen is obstructed.[1] In adults, approximately 90% of all primary tumors of the trachea are malignant, in contrast to 10% to 30% in children. The incidence of tracheal malignancies is about 0.1 in every 100,000 persons per year, corresponding to approximately 0.2% of all tumors of the respiratory tract and to 0.02% to 0.04% of all malignant tumors. Malignancies of the larynx and bronchi are about 40 and 400 times more likely than cancers of the trachea, respectively.[2,3]

Malignant involvement of the trachea predominantly results from direct spread of neighboring tumors, whereas primary tracheal malignancies are usually rare. Compared with the bronchus and lung, their incidence is lower due to the limited surface area epithelium, greater mucociliary stream, and more laminar flow. Normally the trachea is lined by columnar ciliated respiratory epithelium, which has both mucinous and nonmucinous cells. Most of the tracheal neoplasms, both benign and malignant, are squamous rather than mucinous or glandular, thus reflecting a conversion of the epithelium to squamous. This is most likely due to the influence of smoking. The glandular neoplasms are similar to lung and salivary glands. In general, because most of these tumors are obstructing, they are detected early. Squamous cell carcinoma and adenoid cystic carcinoma make up about two-thirds of adult PTT.[4] A heterogeneous group of benign and malignant tumors accounts for the remaining third of tracheal neoplasms.

A listing of these rarer tumors is as follows.

Disclosure: The authors have nothing to disclose.
[a] Department of Surgery, Albany Medical College, 43 New Scotland Avenue, Albany, NY 12208, USA;
[b] Department of Surgery, St. Peter's Hospital, 315 New Scotland Avenue, Albany, NY 12208, USA
* Corresponding author. 18 Burton Lane, Albany, NY 12211.
E-mail address: moores.darroch@gmail.com

Thorac Surg Clin 28 (2018) 149–154
https://doi.org/10.1016/j.thorsurg.2018.01.003
1547-4127/18/© 2018 Elsevier Inc. All rights reserved.

Benign

- Squamous papilloma (multiple or solitary)
- Pleomorphic adenoma
- Granular cell tumor
- Fibrous histiocytoma
- Leiomyoma
- Chondroma
- Chondroblastoma
- Schwannoma
- Paraganglioma
- Hemangioendothelioma
- Vascular malformations

Intermediate

- Carcinoid
- Mucoepidermoid
- Plexiform neurofibroma
- Pseudosarcoma
- Malignant fibrous histocytoma

Malignant

- Adenocarcinoma
- Adenosquamous carcinoma
- Small cell carcinoma
- Atypical carcinoid
- Melanoma
- Chondrosarcoma
- Spindle cell sarcoma
- Rhabdomyosarcoma

SQUAMOUS EPITHELIUM TUMORS
Squamous Cell Carcinoma

Squamous cell carcinoma (**Fig. 1**) is one of the most frequent PTT, comprising about one-third of all tracheal neoplasms. Several variants of squamous cell carcinoma of the hypopharynx, larynx, and trachea are mentioned, including verrucous carcinoma, basaloid carcinoma, papillary

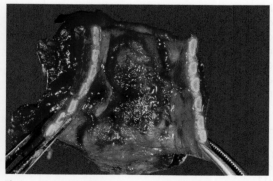

Fig. 1. Extensive squamous cell carcinoma of the lower intrathoracic trachea. Note the typical ulcerated surface of the tumor.

carcinoma, spindle-cell carcinoma, acantholytic carcinoma, and adenosquamous carcinoma. They are much less likely to happen in the trachea as compared with larynx or lung (75 and 180 times, respectively). Smoking is common in most patients. They are more likely in the posterior wall of the lower third. Macroscopically, tracheal squamous cell carcinoma usually grows as a polypoid and frequently ulcerative mass, projecting into the lumen of the trachea. In symptomatic stages, most of these lesions are easily detectable by bronchoscopy. Histologically these tumors are characterized by more or less well-defined squamous differentiation, with or without keratinization.[5] The association with cigarette smoking may lead to metachronous or synchronous lesions of the oropharynx, the larynx, or the lungs.

Squamous Papilloma and Papillomatosis

Squamous papillomas of the trachea are rare benign tumors composed of stratified squamous epithelium with acantholysis and papillomatosis supported by fibrovascular core. They are multiple and recurrent or solidly exophytic growths into the tracheal lumen. In terms of the biology, squamous papillomas of the trachea are often associated with upper posterior laryngeal and all lower bronchial involvement. The patient presents with stridor, wheezing, dyspnea, chest pain, or hemoptysis. Lung parenchyma is affected in about 1% of cases, most of them complicated by necrosis cavitation or pneumonia. Human papilloma virus is a known cause of this tumor, and different types are detected.[6] Squamous cell carcinoma may develop in squamous papillomas, although malignancy is rare in papillomatosis.[7]

Adenocarcinoma

Although the most common lung malignancy, adenocarcinomas are usually located in the lung periphery away from he central airways. Infrequently, they can arise as a primary tracheal tumor. When adenocarcinoma does involve the trachea, it is usually secondary to direct extension from an adjacent tumor or malignant mediastinal lymph node. Adenocarcinomas (**Fig. 2**) affect both sexes mostly in the fifth to eighth decades of life. Presentation is often obstructive. Gross adenocarcinomas are bulky tumors that may bulge into the lumen but may also invade through the tracheal wall into adjacent structures. Microscopically most of these are mucin producing. They form glands with epithelial cells containing large vesicular nuclei and prominent nucleoli. Differential diagnoses include adenoid cystic carcinoma, mucoepidermoid carcinoma, and secondary involvement of trachea from

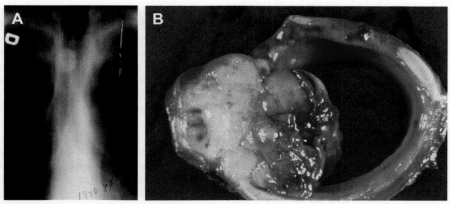

Fig. 2. Adenocarcinoma of the trachea. (*A*) Air tomogram showing an obstructive lesion located over the right tracheal wall. (*B*) Resected specimen showing the tumor invading the membranous trachea.

other primaries. This may include direct invasion from thyroid carcinomas and adenocarcinomas of proximal bronchi extending up to the trachea.[8]

Large Cell Undifferentiated Carcinoma

Large cell undifferentiated carcinomas are very rare, and usually a diagnosis is made by exclusion of squamous cell carcinoma and adenocarcinoma.

NEUROENDOCRINE TUMORS

These neoplasms comprise the spectrum of low-grade typical carcinoids to high-grade neuroendocrine tumors. These tumors are much less frequent in trachea than bronchi probably because of the scarcity of Kulchitsky cells in the trachea. Bronchopulmonary neuroendocrine tumors are classified into low-grade typical carcinoid, intermediate-grade atypical carcinoid, and high-grade carcinoid categories of large cell neuroendocrine carcinomas and small cell carcinomas.[9] In general, like all tracheal tumors, they are rare.

Typical and Atypical Carcinoid Tumors

Carcinoid tumors (**Fig. 3**) are low-grade malignant neoplasms of neuroendocrine cells. They are divided into typical and atypical subtypes with the latter possessing more malignant histologic and atypical features.[10] Carcinoid tumors usually have a main polypoid intraluminal component with the smooth or yellow-tan or pink surface. Occasionally they can be entirely confined to the polyp and have only minor growth in the lamina propria of the tracheal wall. Atypical carcinoids may be more infiltrative through the wall, sometimes with areas of necrosis and hemorrhage. Local lymph metastasis is frequently seen in atypical carcinoids. Microscopically both typical and atypical carcinoids show the so-called neuroendocrine look, which is an organoid

pattern of uniform epithelial cells with a finely granular chromatin pattern, inconspicuous nuclei, and moderate eosinophilic cytoplasm. Atypical carcinoids have coarser chromatin pattern with more prominent nucleoli. It is well known that atypical carcinoids are cytologically more atypical with a high mitotic rate and necrosis. The criteria of separation from typical carcinoids have been challenging. Atypical carcinoid tumors are characterized by a mitotic rate of 2-10 on high-power fields or foci of coagulative necrosis. They are either punctate or large and infarct like. Typical carcinoids are often delimited and have a broad front of invasion. Atypical carcinoids are more likely to have tongues of invasion into the tracheal wall. Vascular and lymphatic invasions are common with atypical carcinoids. Differential diagnoses include small cell carcinoma and undifferentiated large cell carcinoma.

Large Cell Neuroendocrine Carcinoma

Large cell neuroendocrine carcinoma is a high-grade neuroendocrine tumor, which can be mistaken for a carcinoid or atypical carcinoid but

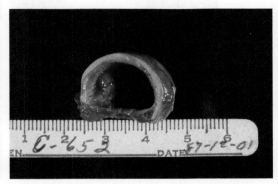

Fig. 3. Atypical carcinoid tumor originating from the left main bronchus and extending to the carina.

has a worse prognosis. Large cell neuroendocrine carcinomas are extremely rare.[11] Microscopically they show neuroendocrine features and need to be differentiated from atypical carcinoids. Small cell carcinomas are sometimes difficult to differentiate particularly when the cells are large or when the biopsies are small and crushed. That prognosis is worse compared with atypical carcinoids.

Small Cell Carcinoma

Small cell carcinomas are extremely rare. When there is extensive paratracheal small cell carcinoma, it may be difficult to differentiate where the tumor arose. They fall within the spectrum of neuroendocrine tumors.

SALIVARY GLAND–TYPE TUMORS

The minor salivary glands existing in the mucous membranes of the head and neck extend downwards as the submucosal glands in the trachea. Therefore, they are subject to most of the so-called salivary gland–type tumors that involve the salivary glands in the head and neck with only a few exceptions. However, the frequency of such tumors is much less in the trachea compared with in the head and neck.

Pleomorphic Adenoma (Mixed Tumor)

Pleomorphic adenoma (mixed tumor) can rarely arise in the tracheobronchial tree. They are most commonly seen in the upper third of the trachea followed by the middle and lower thirds.[8] Typically they are polypoidal, intraluminal masses causing varying degrees of obstruction. Microscopically pleomorphic adenoma is relatively well circumscribed but without a capsule. It consists of a mixture of epithelial cells, myoepithelial cells, and stroma. The epithelial components form sheaths, ducts, trabeculae, and a small nest of cells with vesicular nuclei and small to moderate amounts of cytoplasm. Foci of squamous differentiation may be seen. These areas merge with alternating areas of spindled and stellate cells in myxoid, hyaline, or chondral myxoid stroma. Differential diagnosis includes other salivary-type tumors such as adenoid cystic carcinoma and mucoid epidermoid carcinoma. These tumors have a good prognosis.

Mucous Gland Adenoma

Mucous gland adenoma is a benign tumor of the salivary gland type. It arises in seromucous glands of the tracheobronchial tree. It is characterized by cystlike dilated mucous-filled glands, hence the term mucous gland adenoma. The major differential diagnosis is mucoid epidermoid carcinoma.

Mucoid Epidermoid Carcinoma

Mucoid epidermoid carcinoma is a malignant salivary gland–type tumor (Fig. 4) arising from submucosal glands off the trachea. It is usually rare and

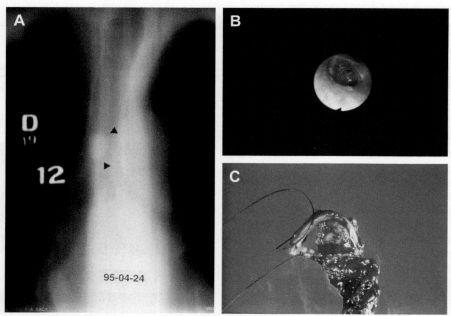

Fig. 4. Tracheal mucoepidermoid carcinoma. (*A*) Air tomogram showing the tumor located in the lower part of the trachea. (*B*) Bronchoscopic view of the tumor. (*C*) Resected specimen.

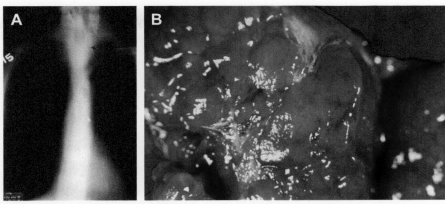

Fig. 5. Thyroid carcinoma invading the trachea. (*A*) Air tomogram showing a large cervicothoracic mass displacing the trachea to the left. (*B*) Resected thyroid carcinoma. In this case, the trachea was invaded but not resected.

affects the trachea even less often than bronchi. These tumors grow as a polypoid tan-gray to pink endotracheal mass. Rarely invasion through the trachea into adventitia is seen in high-grade tumors. Microscopically it is characterized by a variable mix of mucus-secreting cells, squamous cells, and cells of intermediate type.[12] Mucin-producing cells are scattered. Anaplastic features are absent, and the tumor is generally classified as low grade. Differential diagnosis includes squamous cell carcinoma, adenocarcinoma, other salivary gland–type tumors, carcinoid tumor, and mucous gland adenoma.

The most important type of salivary gland-like tumor is the adenoid cystic tumor of the trachea. It is described in detail separately.

Metastatic Tumors of the Trachea

Secondary involvement of the trachea occurs as a direct invasion of adjacent organs, such as larynx, thyroid (**Fig. 5**), esophagus, mediastinal structures, and rarely due to metastases. This is in stark contrast to the bronchial tree, which most commonly receives metastases from distant primaries. Histologically most of the tumors have a subepithelial location with some extending deep into the tracheal wall and even surrounding soft tissue. The overlying epithelium is hyperplastic or ulcerated.

SUMMARY

Overall, tracheal tumors are rare but present early because they tend to be obstructive. Papilloma is the most frequent benign tracheal tumor. Squamous cell carcinomas followed by adenoid cystic carcinomas are the most frequent malignant tracheal cancers and comprise almost two-thirds of all known cases. There is no universally accepted and replicable staging system for these cancers.

REFERENCES

1. Eschapasse H, Gaillard J, Henry E, et al. Neoplastic tracheal stenosis. Int Surg 1982;67:221–7.
2. Honings J, Gaissert HA, van der Heijden HF, et al. Clinical aspects and treatment of primary tracheal malignancies. Acta Otolaryngol 2010;130:763–72.
3. Honings J, van Dijck JA, Verhagen AF, et al. Incidence and treatment of tracheal cancer: a nationwide study in the Netherlands. Ann Surg Oncol 2007;14:968–76.
4. Macchiarini P. Primary tracheal tumours. Lancet Oncol 2006;7:83–91.
5. Heffner DK. Diseases of the trachea. In: Barnes L, editor. Surgical pathology of the head and neck. 2nd edition. New York: Marcel Dekker; 2001. p. 602–31.
6. Popper HH, Wirsberger G, Juttner-smoll FM, et al. The predictive value of human papilloma virus (HPV) typing in the prognosis of bronchial squamous cell papillomas. Histopathology 1992; 21:323–30.
7. Runckel D, Kessler S. Bronchogenic squamous carcinoma in non-irradiated juvenile laryngotracheal papillomatosis. Am J Surg Pathol 1980;4: 293–6.
8. Zirkin HJ, Tovi F. Tracheal carcinoma presenting as a thyroid tumor. J Surg Oncol 1985;26:268–71.
9. Colby TV, Koss MN, Travis WD. Carcinoid and other neuroendocrine tumors. In: Atlas of tumors pathology. Tumors of the lower respiratory tract. Washington, DC: Armed Forces Institute of Pathology; 1995. p. 283–317.
10. Arrigoni MG, Woolner LB, Bernatz PE. Atypical carcinoid tumors of the lung. J Thorac Cardiovasc Surg 1972;64:413–21.

11. Tartour E, Caillou B, Tenebaum F, et al. Neuroendocrine tumor of the trachea of the intermediate type. Value of its individualization. Presse Med 1992;21: 1905–8.

12. Schanmugarten K. Histological typing of tumors of the upper respiratory tract and ear, vol. 60. Berlin: World Health Organization; 1991. p. 1346–62.

Tuberculosis and Other Granulomatous Diseases of the Airway

Rajan Santosham, MS, MCh, FRCS[a],*,
Jean Deslauriers, MD, FRCS(C), CM[b]

KEYWORDS

- Granuloma • Tuberculosis • Histoplasmosis • Wegener granulomatosis

KEY POINTS

- Granulomatous diseases of the airway are challenging lesions to diagnose and effectively manage because of their rarity and occurrence in different forms, each with unique clinical and radiological characteristics.
- Granulomatous diseases of the airway are not as common as granulomatous diseases involving the lung or other organs.
- Tuberculosis is still a major concern in underdeveloped countries, whereas histoplasmosis is relatively common in eastern and central United States.
- Most granulomatous diseases of the airway can be effectively managed conservatively with drug treatment and repeated airway dilatation.
- Surgical resection may be beneficial in cases presenting with localized airway obstruction or severe hemoptysis.

INTRODUCTION

Granulomas consist of compact aggregates of histiocytes (macrophages) known as "epithelioid histiocytes" because they have elongated cell borders and sole-shaped nuclei as opposed are to what is seen in "ordinary histiocytes," which have well-defined cell borders and round or oval nuclei.[1] The granulomatous inflammatory reaction itself relates to cell-mediated immunity and delayed hypersensitivity and represents the last line of pulmonary defenses. Pathologically, granulomas are characterized by the accumulation of blood-derived macrophages, epithelioid histiocytes, plasma cells, and multinucleated giant cells, representing fused macrophages. T lymphocytes can also be found around the periphery of granulomas. Granulomas can be either infectious or noninfectious in origin and necrotizing or nonnecrotizing.

Granulomatous diseases of the airway are often difficult to diagnose because they can occur in different forms, each with unique clinical and radiological features. Although airway involvement–related symptoms may be the initial clinical manifestation of disease, such involvement is, in most cases, indicative of a more generalized illness. The diagnosis of airway granulomatous disease can generally be established through radiographic and bronchoscopic examinations, whereas management can vary from observation alone to specific drug treatment, repeated airway

Disclosure: The authors have nothing to disclose.
a Department of Thoracic Surgery, Santosham Chest Hospital, 155, Egmore High Road, Egmore, Chennai 600008, India; b Laval University, 6364, Chemin Royal, Saint-Laurent-de-l'Île-d'Orléans, Quebec City, Québec G0A3Z0, Canada
* Corresponding author.
E-mail address: drrajansantosham@yahoo.com

thoracic.theclinics.com

dilatation, or surgical resection in cases presenting with localized and/or symptomatic airway obstruction or life-threatening complications, such as massive hemoptysis.

The 3 most common granulomatous airway disease processes that are likely to have an impact for thoracic surgeons are tuberculosis (MTB), histoplasmosis with secondary broncholithiasis, and Wegener granulomatosis (WG).

AIRWAY TUBERCULOSIS

MTB (*Mycobacterium tuberculosis*), called phthisis or the Great Plague, was the disease that initiated the birth of thoracic surgery near the end of the nineteenth century. It was one of the few remaining unsolved epidemics, its incidence having been accelerated by the "Industrial Revolution" throughout Europe with population shifts toward the cities, overcrowding, and people living in generally poor hygienic conditions. At the time, it was considered to be the most common cause of death worldwide.

For a long time, MTB was considered to be a disease occurring almost exclusively in underdeveloped countries. This concept is, however, no longer true because a significant number of cases are now diagnosed in industrial countries, a phenomenon that relates to an increased incidence of the AIDS syndrome, which predisposes to MTB, an ever-increasing geriatric population, and, finally, the occurrence of multiple-drug-resistant tuberculosis. In industrial countries, for instance, most MTB cases occur in the elderly population, whereas in developing countries, 80% of cases occur in people younger than 60 years of age.

Airway MTB can be secondary to direct implant of tuberculous bacilli from pulmonary lesions containing numerous bacilli into the airway, or it can occur, perhaps more commonly, in relation to local spreading along peribronchial lymphatic channels.[2,3] Isolated airway MTB is a much rarer entity that can, at times, be misinterpreted as being a primary airway neoplasm.[4]

The 4 commonest patterns of tuberculous airway disease that are pertinent to thoracic surgeons are those of (1) extrinsic airway obstruction by tuberculous lymph nodes, (2) endobronchial and endotracheal MTB with secondary stenosis, (3) tracheoesophageal (TEFs) or bronchoesophageal fistulas (BEFs), and (4) the so-called middle lobe syndrome (**Table 1**).

Extrinsic Airway Obstruction by Tuberculous Lymph Nodes

Although enlarged mediastinal nodes are common in patients with pulmonary MTB, it is only in a

Table 1
Number of cases of airway tuberculosis seen by one of the authors (R.J.) at the Santosham Chest Hospital in Chennai, India over the past 20 y (Rajan Santosham, unpublished data)

Predominant Pattern of Disease	No. of Cases
Extrinsic obstruction by tuberculous lymph nodes	124
Endotracheal/endobronchial MTB with secondary stenosis	84
TEF/BEF	26
Middle lobe syndrome	84
Total	318

minority of cases (2%–5%) that they will cause airway compression severe enough to be symptomatic and/or require specific therapeutic interventions. Presenting symptoms are usually cough and stridor, which may be mistakenly attributed to asthma or even bronchogenic carcinoma (**Fig. 1**). In extreme cases, the involved nodes can even unload caseum into the tracheal or bronchial lumen, resulting in sudden respiratory deterioration or even death. Because of their yet poorly developed cartilaginous support, children are more susceptible to mediastinal lymph node compression than are the adults. Because thoracic imaging may not demonstrate clear-cut pulmonary involvement in this subset of patients, the preferred diagnostic method is that of bronchoscopy, which will confirm airway tuberculous granulomatous involvement through either endoluminal biopsies or positive bronchial washings.

Extrinsic airway obstruction is usually responsive to medical therapy, particularly that of corticosteroids. In the rare instance where the obstruction becomes clinically significant, surgical decompression may be necessary. Such operations are usually carried out through a right posterolateral thoracotomy and consist of nodal incision with either aspiration or curettage of nodal contents. Because some of these lymph nodes may contain a liquefied core, bronchoscopic debridement and drainage are sometimes possible.

Endobronchial and Endotracheal Tuberculosis with Secondary Stenosis

Endobronchial or endotracheal MTB (active or sequelae) is seen in approximately 10% to 20% of patients with pulmonary MTB,[5] and it can lead to cicatricial stenosis most commonly observed in the distal trachea or main stem bronchi.

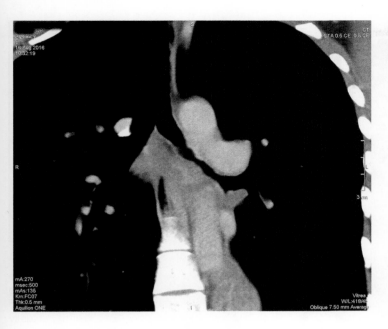

Fig. 1. CT scan showing diffuse narrowing of the left main bronchus secondary to tuberculous lymph nodes. Such a narrowing is often misinterpreted as being secondary to carcinoma.

Classically, these patients will present with cough, bronchorrea, and shortness of breath on exertion, and the diagnosis will be made through bronchoscopic examination and biopsies. Sputum analysis and smears are notoriously unreliable in most of those individuals, even in the early stages of disease.

If the condition is diagnosed early, the progression to fixed stenosis can occasionally be prevented by the administration of inhaled or systemic steroids. For well-established long-segment stenosis, surgical resection is usually not possible, and periodic balloon dilatation (**Fig. 2**) with or without stenting of the lesion is the treatment of choice. Short-segment stenosis is, however, best managed by airway resection with primary reconstruction. Pulmonary resection, in either the form of lobectomy, bronchoplastic procedure,[6] or even pneumonectomy, may also be indicated in cases whereby the distal parenchyma is destroyed (destroyed lung) (**Fig. 3**). It is important to remember that such procedures should almost never be done unless the active MTB process is well under control with antituberculous drug treatment.

Tracheoesophageal or Bronchoesophageal Fistulas

TEF or BEF can occasionally be associated with MTB and, in such cases, the fistula results from continuous pressure exerted by scarred posttuberculous mediastinal nodes located between the airway and the esophagus. TEF and BEF most commonly occur at the levels of the distal trachea, main bronchi, and right lower lobe bronchus.

In the acute setting, treatment consists of percutaneous feeding gastrostomy or jejunostomy for food rerouting and antituberculous drug treatment. Interestingly, most fistulas will heal with this type of conservative management. If, however, the fistula persists after a full course of antituberculous treatment, surgical management may become necessary, and correction requires closure of the esophageal defect, segmental airway resection, and tissue interposition.

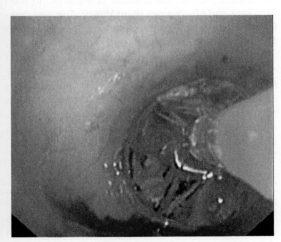

Fig. 2. Balloon dilatation of airway stenosis secondary to MTB.

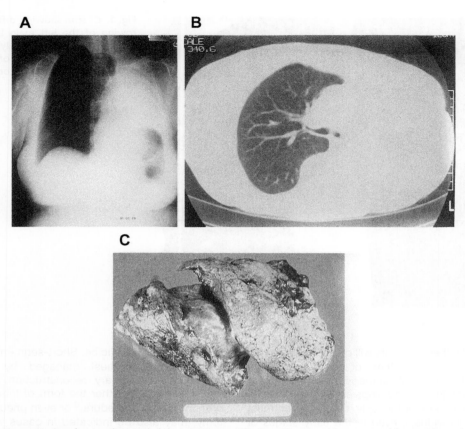

Fig. 3. Posteroanterior chest radiograph (*A*) and CT scan (*B*) of an 80-year-old woman with complete obstruction of the distal left main stem bronchus. Both the radiograph and the scan show complete atelectasis of the left lung. At operation, the lung (*C*) was found to be completely consolidated and had to be removed.

Middle Lobe Syndrome

Isolated atelectasis of the middle lobe is known as the "middle lobe syndrome." It is caused by extrinsic nodal compression, usually of tuberculous origin, on the middle lobe bronchus resulting in chronic postobstructive atelectasis and pneumonitis. Although a similar process could potentially occur anywhere else in either lungs, the middle lobe is particularly susceptible because it has a long and narrow bronchus, which originates at a right angle from the bronchus intermedius. In addition, the middle lobe has no collateral ventilation in individuals with complete fissures. Symptoms are usually those of recurrent pulmonary infection, and it is always important to rule out obstruction by a malignant neoplasm, which could produce the same radiologic appearance and symptoms.

Once the diagnosis of benign disease has been confirmed, and if the patient is symptomatic, surgical resection of the middle lobe is generally curative. No surgery is necessary for patients with asymptomatic middle lobe syndrome.

HISTOPLASMOSIS AND SECONDARY BRONCHOLITHIASIS

Histoplasmosis is a fungal infection caused by the dimorphic fungus "Histoplasma capsulatum." In the United States, the disease is endemic in the Midwest and Mississippi River Valley. The reasons for this particular geographic distribution are thought to include the moderate climate, humidity, and soil characteristics in those areas. Although millions of people are infected with this fungus, relatively few will present with clinical signs or symptoms of the disease. In its chronic phase, histoplasmosis can affect major airways through mediastinal granulomas externally compressing the tracheobronchial tree or frankly eroding into them.

Broncholithiasis

Broncholithiasis is a rare condition in which one or more calcified nodes (broncholiths) are found within or have eroded through the tracheobronchial lumen causing clinical symptoms and radiographic abnormalities. This definition can be expanded to include cases in which peritracheobronchial calcified lymph nodes distort the airway without actual intrusion into their lumen.

Although most broncholiths are secondary to histoplasmosis, they can also result from mycobacterial granulomatous lymphadenitis, silicosis, or both.[7,8] Their pathogenesis relates to the precipitation of calcium salts during the healing process of the fungal infection. They are made of 85% to 95% calcium phosphate and 7% to 10% calcium carbonate. Because of the repetitive motion of respiratory movements, heartbeats, and deglutition, these calcified nodes eventually cause pressure atrophy of the tracheobronchial wall, erosion, and migration into their lumen.[9–11] They can also cause bronchial narrowing with distal infection, bronchiectasis, and atelectasis. They can finally penetrate adjacent blood vessels, causing hemoptysis, or adjacent structures, such as the esophagus, causing tracheobronchoesophageal fistulas.

Broncholithiasis has a predilection for the right lung, particularly the bronchus intermedius. It occurs equally in both men and women and at any age. Symptoms can be quite variable, and, in general, they depend on the physical characteristics of the broncholith, such as its size, location, whether it is mobile or fixed, and its relationship with the adjacent airway. The most common symptoms are those of chronic and unproductive cough due to airway irritation, lithoptysis (expectoration of stones), hemoptysis, purulent sputum, and, on occasion, symptoms related to a tracheobronchoesophageal fistula.

The diagnosis of broncholithiasis is most commonly based on radiographic findings as well as bronchoscopic observation of the broncholith itself (**Fig. 4**). A conventional chest radiograph may show calcified hilar nodes, whereas a multiplane reformation helical computed tomographic (CT) scan will easily document the calcified lymph nodes and whether they are endobronchial or peribronchial. CT scanning will also depict the exact morphology of the broncholith as well as its relationship with pulmonary blood vessels and other adjacent mediastinal structures. Bronchoscopy may show the stone within the tracheobronchial lumen or embedded in its wall. It may also show airway obstruction by a hard calcified mass, bleeding, mucosal inflammation, or sometimes the site of a tracheobronchoesophageal fistula. Bronchoscopy is also helpful to rule out an airway neoplasm.

Broncholithiasis can be managed by observation alone, bronchoscopic broncholithiectomy, or surgery depending on the characteristics of the broncholith. If the broncholith is small, not associated with significant symptoms or complications, observation alone may be all that is necessary. The exact role of endoscopic removal is controversial, although most agree that it can be attempted if the stone is small and mobile with minimal fixation (loose broncholithiasis),[12,13] if it is proximal enough to allow its grasping through the bronchoscope, and if it is not contiguous with blood vessels. These procedures should always, however, be done with great caution because the visible endoluminal mass may extend beyond the airway and be densely adherent to the adjacent pulmonary artery.

Surgery is generally indicated for complications of the condition, including intractable cough, severe or recurring hemoptysis, airway obstruction, or tracheobronchoesophageal or vascular fistula. On occasion, surgery may also be indicated for the treatment of complications related to failed attempts at bronchoscopic removal of the broncholith! Surgical options include anatomic pulmonary resection or broncholithectomy with or without bronchoplasty. In general, the rule of thumb is to remove all diseased lung and nodes while attempting to preserve normal lung. These procedures are always technically difficult owing to the dense contiguous fibrotic reaction and likely adherence of the granuloma to the airway. On occasion, it is advisable to leave behind the capsule of the calcified mass (decompression by incision and curettage) in order to prevent serious airway or vascular damage.

The long-term prognosis after surgery is good,[11,14,15] although recurrence of broncholithiasis can occur in 15% to 20% of patients. Antifungal treatment has virtually no role in the management of isolated broncholithiasis.

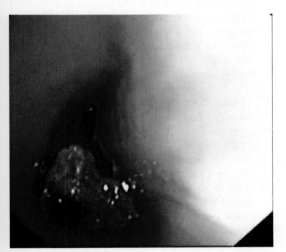

Fig. 4. Typical bronchoscopic image of a broncholith.

WEGENER GRANULOMATOSIS

WG is characterized by disseminated necrotizing granulomatous inflammation and necrotizing vasculitis mainly affecting the small arteries, arterioles, capillaries, and venules of the kidneys and airways. Cutaneous, musculoskeletal, and ocular involvement can also occur, whereas cardiac and central nervous systems are seldom afflicted. Airway involvement, both upper and lower, occurs in 15% to 55% of patients, and it is one of the major features of the disease.[16] Although the exact cause of WG is unknown, the coexistence of granulomatous inflammation and vasculitis suggests that delayed hypersensitivity and antigen-antibody or immunologic reactions mediated by immune complexes are occurring.[17]

Involvement of the respiratory mucosa can occur all along the upper and lower airway, and in about 25% of patients, it will be the only manifestation of disease.[16] Respiratory involvement (airway, lung) is also an essential requirement to make the diagnosis of WG. WG is more common in young individuals and in women, and airway pathologic findings include nasal cartilage necrosis, nasal stenosis, subglottic stricture as well as stenosis of the trachea and main bronchi. Alveolar infiltrates as well as granulomatous lung masses can also be observed.

Symptoms related to upper airway involvement include rhinorrhea, sinusitis, nasopharyngeal ulcerations, and serous otitis media, whereas those related to lower airway involvement include cough, stridor, and hemoptysis, which, on occasion, can be quite severe. The diagnosis of WG can usually be confirmed at bronchoscopy, which is also useful for follow-up, or through open lung biopsy.

Subglottic strictures are, in most cases, the presenting features of the disease,[16] and they are usually unresponsive to immunosuppressive therapy.[18] For such patients, endoscopic treatment is a good alternative, but other possible causes of subglottic strictures, such as postintubation strictures or idiopathic strictures, must first be ruled out. Endoscopic therapy options include repeated balloon dilatation, dilatation through the use of metal dilators, laser therapy, or placement of an endoprosthesis. In some cases, an emergency tracheostomy may have to be done and, for localized lesions, surgical laryngotracheal resection and reconstruction may be required.[19]

For most cases, however, an oral single dose of cyclophosphamide should be considered as first-line treatment because it will often be associated with short- and long-term remissions. For rapidly progressive disease, it may be better to initiate treatment with intravenous cyclophosphamide (2–3 mg/kg/d) for a few days followed by oral treatment (1–2 mg/kg/d). With the increased life expectancy of patients with WG being on cyclophosphamide treatment, endotracheobronchial complications are likely to be seen with increasing frequency, thus the need for careful and prolonged follow-up in these individuals.

SUMMARY

The role of the thoracic surgeon in managing granulomatous diseases of the airway has decreased significantly since the advent of effective medications beginning with the discovery of anti-tuberculous drugs in the late 1940s. The recent resurgence of resistant forms of disease or of immunocompromised hosts has made these diseases, however, more common, especially in underdeveloped countries. When patients fail medical treatment or present life-threatening complications, such as hemoptysis or airway obstruction, surgery remains a very effective tool in the management of these difficult problems. One of the authors of this essay (R.S.) has reported the practice in India, where MTB is still prevalent (see **Table 1**).

REFERENCES

1. Mukhopadhyay S, Gal AA. Granulomatous lung disease. An approach to the differential diagnosis. Arch Pathol Lab Med 2010;134:667–90.
2. Ip MS, So SY, Lam WK, et al. Endobronchial tuberculosis revisited. Chest 1986;89:727–30.
3. Smith LS, Schillaci RF, Sarlin RF. Endobronchial tuberculosis. serial fiberoptic bronchoscopy and natural history. Chest 1987;91:644–7.
4. Barman S, Khaund G. Primary tuberculosis of upper airway: case report of 3 rare presentation. Indian J Otolaryngol Head Neck Surg 2014;66:208–11.
5. Jokinen K, Palva T, Nuutinen J. Bronchial findings in pulmonary tuberculosis. Clin Otolaryngol 1977;2: 139–48.
6. Kato R, Kakizaki T, Hangai N, et al. Bronchoplastic procedures for tuberculous bronchial stenosis. J Thorac Cardiovasc Surg 1993;106:1118–21.
7. Baum GL, Bernstein L, Schwartz J. Broncholithiasis produced by histoplasmosis. Am Rev Tuberc 1958; 77:162–7.
8. Weed LA, Andersen HA. Etiology of broncholithiasis. Dis Chest 1960;37:270–7.
9. Dixon GF, Donnerberg RL, Schonfeld SA, et al. Advances in the diagnosis and treatment of broncholithiasis. Am Rev Respir Dis 1984;129:1028–30.
10. Bhagavan BS, Rao DRG, Weinberg T. Histoplasmosis producing broncholithiasis. Arch Pathol 1971;91: 577–9.

11. Trastek VF, Pairolero P, Ceithaml EL, et al. Surgical management of broncholithiasis. J Thor Cardiovasc Surg 1985;90:842–8.

12. Menivale F, Deslee G, Vallerand H, et al. Therapeutic management of broncholithiasis. Ann Thorac Surg 2005;79:1774–6.

13. Cole FH, Cole FH Jr, Khandekar A, et al. Management of broncholithiasis: is thoracotomy necessary? Ann Thorac Surg 1986;42:255–7.

14. Faber LP, Jensik RJ, Chawla SK, et al. The surgical implication of broncholithiasis. J Thorac Cardiovasc Surg 1975;70:779–88.

15. Potaris K, iller DL, Trastek VF, et al. Role of surgical resection in broncholithiasis. Ann Thorac Surg 2000; 70:248–52.

16. Rodrigues AJ, Jacomelli M, Baldow RX, et al. Laryngeal and tracheobronchial involvement in Wegener's granulomatosis. Rev Bras Reumatol 2012;52:227–35.

17. Banki F, Wood D. Inflammatory conditions of the airway. In: Patterson GA, Cooper JD, Deslauriers J, et al, editors. Pearson's thoracic and esophageal surgery. Philadelphia: Churchill Livingstone; 2008. p. 294. Chapter 23.

18. Strange C, Halstead L, Baumann M, et al. Subglottic stenosis in Wegener's granulomatosis: development during cyclophosphamide treatment with response to carbon dioxide laser therapy. Thorax 1990;45:300–1.

19. Gluth MB, Shinners PA, Kasperbauer JL. Subglottic stenosis associated with Wegener's granulomatosis. Laryngoscope 2003;113:1304–7.

Tracheobronchomalacia and Expiratory Collapse of Central Airways

Cameron D. Wright, MD

KEYWORDS

• Tracheal surgery • Tracheomalacia • Tracheobronchomalacia

KEY POINTS

- Tracheobronchomalacia is an uncommon acquired cause of central airway collapse.
- Dynamic computed tomographic scan, pulmonary function studies, and functional bronchoscopy are the mainstays of evaluation.
- Tracheobronchoplasty is performed by stabilization of the posterior membranous wall with a stiffening splint material.
- Most patients report an improved quality of life after tracheobronchoplasty.

INTRODUCTION

Tracheobronchomalacia in adults is uncommon and often an incidental finding on a chest computed tomographic (CT) scan done for another reason with mild to moderate airway collapse seen on an expiratory study. These patients just need reassurance. Severe airway collapse (>90%) is rare and usually associated with symptoms such as dyspnea, incessant coughing, inability (or difficulty) raising secretions, and repeated chest infections.[1] These patients are often miserable, and it often takes them a long time to get diagnosed and referred because many clinicians are not familiar with this uncommon disease. If patients are smokers and have associated chronic obstructive pulmonary disease (COPD), it can be very troublesome and challenging to sort out which disease is most important and whether to offer an operation. The author tends to refrain from operating on those with significant COPD unless he is quite convinced that the tracheobronchomalacia is very dominant. The evaluation process starts with a high-quality dynamic chest CT with inspiratory and expiratory views to determine the degree of tracheobronchomalacia and whether it extends to the major bronchi. If severe malacia is found, then an awake functional bronchoscopy is done to verify this and further assess the airway. All airways collapse with a strong cough, and that finding is not diagnostic of tracheobronchomalacia. During quiet breathing with exhalation, if the airway collapses 80% to 90%, then more severe malacia is confirmed. Sometimes coughing will be incited by the opposition of the anterior and posterior walls of the airway. There are 2 anatomic forms of tracheomalacia: the classic soft/weak anterior tracheal cartilages (cartilaginous malacia) with a redundant posterior membranous wall (can be seen with tracheobronchomegaly–Mounier-Kuhn syndrome) and excessive forward displacement of the membranous wall (membranous malacia). Pulmonary function tests are performed to document any other lung abnormality and help assess the risk for thoracotomy. Lung function tests are often relatively normal in the absence of any other pulmonary disease. There is no specific finding on

Disclosure: The author has nothing to disclose.
Division of Thoracic Surgery, Massachusetts General Hospital, Harvard Medical School, Founders 7, 55 Fruit Street, Boston, MA 02114, USA
E-mail address: cdwright@mgh.harvard.edu

thoracic.theclinics.com

pulmonary function studies that is diagnostic of tracheobronchomalacia. Some investigators have advocated a trial of a silicone Y stent in an attempt to document whether symptoms and quality of life are improved with airway stenting as a diagnostic strategy to decide if tracheobronchoplasty would be beneficial.[2] Alternatively, a noncovered metallic stent can be inserted for a short time for a trial of airway stenting.[3] The author has not found this particularly helpful because several patients have not been able to tolerate a stent even for 1 day because of coughing and airway irritation. In addition, mucus plugging of the stent is a not uncommon complication of a temporary stent. In general, the author recommends an operation if severe symptoms match the imaging and bronchoscopic findings of severe expiratory collapse of the airway.

The principle of membranous wall splinting is to stabilize and add rigidity in the case of membranous malacia and to also reconfigure the normal shape of the trachea in the case of cartilaginous malacia (**Fig. 1**). The trachea is typically quite widened with a redundant membranous wall in patients with cartilaginous malacia. Patients with membranous malacia usually have a trachea of normal size (about 2.5 cm from side to side in

the adult), and thus, the membranous wall is not redundant. The posterior membranous wall of the trachea is reinforced with sequential rows of 4-0 mattress sutures placed in a partial thickness fashion. Typically, 4 sutures are placed across the membranous wall with the lateral sutures also catching a small bite of the lateral cartilaginous wall of the trachea (**Fig. 2**). The surgeon needs to estimate the degree of reduction in the width of the membranous wall that will re-create the D shape of the trachea. The reduction in tracheal width can be done by pinching the middle of the membranous wall together and assessing the shape of the cartilaginous trachea until the desired shape and size are achieved. The distance between the lateral walls of the trachea is then measured and used to cut the appropriate size of the stabilizing material. The author's group first used polypropylene mesh for membranous wall stabilization, reasoning it was easy to use and flexible but did not stretch and resisted infection. Most surgeons continue to use it. The author no longer uses it because he has had 2 patients develop late erosion of the mesh into the airway, which created a very challenging late complication with severe granulation tissue and infection in the airway. The author currently uses extra-thick acellular dermis with good medium-term results. He tried polytetrafluoroethylene (PTFE) once, but the patient developed a fluid collection between the

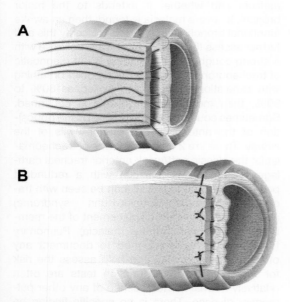

Fig. 1. (*A*) Four sutures are placed across the back wall of the trachea as shown and sutured to a posterior membraneous wall stiffening material. (*B*) When the sutures are tied the membranous wall is plicated and thus made more narrow which reconfigures the shape and collapsibility of the trachea. (*From* Wright CD. Tracheal surgery: posterior splinting tracheoplasty for tracheomalacia. Oper Tech Thorac Cardiovasc Surg 2015;20:42; with permission.)

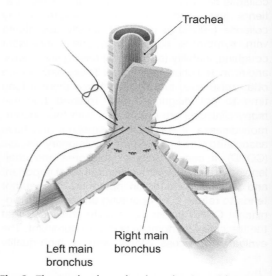

Fig. 2. The tracheobronchoplasty begins with suturing the splinting material at the level of the carina and then works cephalad with 4 mattress sutures for each row. (*From* Wright CD. Tracheal surgery: posterior splinting tracheoplasty for tracheomalacia. Oper Tech Thorac Cardiovasc Surg 2015;20:41; with permission.)

PTFE sheet and the membranous wall that caused obstruction of the airway. Whatever is used must be safe to provide stabilization of the airway for decades but not erode into either the esophagus or the airway. Different sutures have been used for fixing the splinting material to the membranous wall. These sutures include 4-0 polypropylene and polydioxanone (PDS). It is not clear what material is the best suture material to use, permanent or temporary. It is not uncommon when attempting to place partial-thickness sutures that they are actually full thickness into the airway, thus potentially introducing bacteria next to the splint and a foreign body into the airway. PDS eventually dissolves, thus eliminating the issue of foreign body in the airway but potentially would allow the repair to weaken and fall apart with time. The author currently uses PDS with good results but does not have 10-year follow-up.

OPERATION

All patients have a thoracic epidural placed for postoperative pain control. General anesthesia is used, and the patient is intubated with an extra-long wire-reinforced single-lumen endotracheal tube that is positioned with the aid of a bronchoscope in the distal left main bronchus. A double-lumen tube is not used because its large size can interfere with suturing the membranous wall. The patient is placed in the standard left lateral decubitus position and padded appropriately. A high standard right posterolateral thoracotomy is performed in the fourth interspace. The azygous vein is divided, and the mediastinal pleuron is incised over the membranous wall of the trachea and main bronchi. The vagus nerve is preserved. The posterior airway is fully exposed from the thoracic inlet to the main bronchi. The lateral and anterior aspects of the trachea are not dissected out to avoid damage to the recurrent laryngeal nerves and to avoid devascularizing the trachea. If the main bronchi are involved, then the dissection extends down to the right bronchus intermedius and down the left main bronchus to the upper lobe takeoff.

Once the posterior airway is exposed, the splinting material must be cut and fashioned to the appropriate width and length. If the main bronchi need to be splinted as well, either separate strips can be cut for each main bronchus (usually 1 cm for the left main bronchus and 1.5 cm for the right main bronchus) or a Y-shaped strip can be cut out of wider material so there is one continuous strip. The author now prefers to make his splint as a Y because it seems somewhat easier. The repair is started by anchoring the distal tracheal end at the carina with a stitch at the carinal spur and in the middle of the main bronchi and at the lateral edges of the tracheobronchial angle. Middle sutures are placed in a mattress fashion through the splint, then a partial thickness bite through the membranous wall, and then back through the splint again. These sutures are placed one-third and two-thirds of the way across the membranous wall. The lateral stitches catch the junction of the membranous wall and the cartilaginous wall for extra strength. The author places all 4 stitches across one row, each individually snapped and then organized on the drapes, and holds off on tying them. The author then places the next row of 4 sutures and then ties the preceding row. The author finds it easier to place the stitches and position the splint for optimal suturing if the preceding row is not tied down. Each row is placed about 5 to 7 mm apart, and the repair is continued until the thoracic inlet area is reached. The malacia almost always stops at the thoracic inlet so there is no need to try and expose the trachea in the neck. Once the trachea is done, the bronchi are done next, if required. The author does the right first and then the left. The left is the most difficult because of poor exposure deep in the mediastinum and the presence of the endotracheal tube. The cuff should be temporarily deflated and ventilation stopped when suturing the left main bronchus so the cuff is not inadvertently punctured.

If possible, sutures should be partial thickness in the airway. However, practically speaking, it is not uncommon to find at the end during surveillance bronchoscopy that there are several (out of dozens) inadvertent sites of suture penetration. The author has not gone back and removed those and replaced them because it would be very challenging to identify each full-thickness suture. The completed repair is seen in **Fig. 3**.

Surveillance bronchoscopy at the conclusion of the procedure is done by pulling the endotracheal tube back to the proximal trachea and inspecting the result of the repair during inspiration and expiration. Any significant residual abnormality or inadvertent issues (such as narrowing of the right upper lobe bronchus if the main and intermedius is splinted) should be identified and corrected at this time rather than postoperatively. A single chest tube is placed and the thoracotomy is closed in the routine fashion. Patients are extubated in the operating room and often require some temporary positive pressure support until they are fully awake. Observation in the intensive care unit is usually advised because these patients

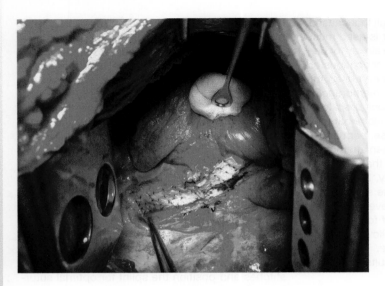

Fig. 3. Completed tracheobronchoplasty seen through a right posterior thoracotomy.

often have airway issues and difficulty clearing secretions for a few days. Care is otherwise routine as for a major thoracotomy.

DISCUSSION

Patients who are properly selected and have a good anatomic result often mention early in the postoperative period that they feel they are better despite the presence of a painful thoracotomy incision.[4–6] The morbidity is usually pulmonary in nature and runs the gamut of atelectasis, sputum retention, pneumonia, and respiratory failure. Mortality after operation is quite rare. Quality-of-life measures are improved in most patients, and functional testing with the 6-minute walk test also demonstrates improvement in most patients.[5,6] Pulmonary function tests usually do not measurably improve. Certainly, one of the problems in evaluating these patients (either preoperatively or postoperatively) is the subjective nature of their symptoms and how they perceive their respiratory health. In the end, the goal is a satisfied patient despite the lack of a quantifiable metric. Indeed, postoperative surveys of patients have reported that most patients are improved and satisfied with the results of a tracheoplasty.[4–6] Rarely, patients may return with symptoms of tracheomalacia again after operation and may have isolated cervical tracheomalacia. Cervical tracheoplasty

has been reported to improve patients with that unusual condition.[7]

REFERENCES

1. Murgu SD, Colt HG. Tracheobronchomalacia and excessive dynamic airway collapse. Respirology 2006;11:388–406.
2. Ernst A, Majid A, Feller-Kopman D, et al. Airway stabilization with silicone stents for treating adult tracheobronchomalacia: a prospective observational trial. Chest 2007;132:609–16.
3. Majid A, Alape D, Kheir F, et al. Short-term use of uncovered self-expanding metallic airway stents for severe expiratory central airway collapse. Respiration 2016;92:389–96.
4. Wright CD, Grillo HC, Hammoud ZT, et al. Tracheoplasty for expiratory collapse of the airways. Ann Thorac Surg 2005;80:259–66.
5. Gangadharan SP, Bakhos CT, Majid A, et al. Technical aspects and outcomes of tracheobronchoplasty for severe tracheobronchomalacia. Ann Thorac Surg 2011;91:1574–81.
6. Buitrago DH, Wilson JL, Parikh M, et al. Current concepts in severe adult tracheobronchomalacia: evaluation and treatment. J Thorac Dis 2017;9:E57–66.
7. Wilson JL, Folch E, Kent MS, et al. Posterior mesh tracheoplasty for cervical tracheomalacia: a novel trachea-preserving technique. Ann Thorac Surg 2016;101:372–4.

Surgery of the Proximal Airway

Contemporary Management of Idiopathic Laryngotracheal Stenosis

Laura Donahoe, MD[a,b], Shaf Keshavjee, MD[a,*]

KEYWORDS

- Pearson procedure • Idiopathic laryngotracheal stenosis • Subglottic tracheal resection
- Airway reconstruction

KEY POINTS

- Idiopathic subglottic stenosis is a rare diagnosis affecting predominantly women, whose etiology is yet to be understood.
- Endoscopic treatment can be successful for some patients with idiopathic subglottic stenosis, yet recurrence rates are high despite multimodal therapy.
- Subglottic tracheal resection with synchronous laryngeal resection and preservation of the recurrent laryngeal nerves can provide excellent and durable outcomes for patients with idiopathic subglottic stenosis.

INTRODUCTION

Idiopathic subglottic stenosis (ISS) was first described in the 1970s,[1] and is a rare but well-described indication for airway intervention and subglottic tracheal resection. As described, ISS is a diagnosis of exclusion, made after ruling out other common causes of stenosis (**Box 1**).

Controversy exists regarding the optimal treatment for ISS; thus, it is imperative that the diagnosis is correct and all other etiologies are ruled out by history, blood work (eg, antineutrophilic cytoplasmic antibody for granulomatosis with polyangiitis, angiotensin-converting enzyme for sarcoidosis) and imaging. These patients are typically women aged 20 to 60 years, with a typical history of insidious onset dyspnea and noisy breathing that often lasts months to years before diagnosis.[2,3] Often, these patients are treated for other conditions or misdiagnosed as having "asthma" before the diagnosis of ISS. Although most of these patients generally do not have a history of prolonged intubation, many have a history of a short intubation for a surgical procedure.[3–6] There are no data to support that short periods of intubation (such as for elective surgical procedures) contribute to the development of the stenosis. As an anecdotal observation, short stature women who develop postintubation subglottic stenosis likely experience trauma to the subglottic airway because they have a smaller trachea; the clinical tendency is to use a standard sized endotracheal tube such as a size 7.0 or 7.5 for routine intubation, which is actually too large for these patient. Also, gastroesophageal reflux disease has been postulated as a potential causative or contributing factor in the development of ISS. There are no definitive data supporting this suggestion, however, and many patients presenting with ISS have no history of gastroesophageal reflux disease, although it may contribute to the development of ISS in some patients.[6–8] Because

Disclosure: The authors have nothing to disclose.
a Division of Thoracic Surgery, Toronto General Hospital, 200 Elizabeth Street, 9N-946, Toronto, Ontario M5G 2C4, Canada; b Division of Thoracic Surgery, Toronto General Hospital, 200 Elizabeth Street, 9N-985, Toronto, Ontario M5G 2C4, Canada
* Corresponding author.
E-mail address: shaf.keshavjee@uhn.ca

Thorac Surg Clin 28 (2018) 167–175
https://doi.org/10.1016/j.thorsurg.2018.01.011
1547-4127/18/© 2018 Elsevier Inc. All rights reserved.

Box 1
Causes of subglottic tracheal stenosis

Postintubation

Trauma

Inhalational burns

Radiation

Collagen vascular diseases (including granulomatosis with polyangiitis, sarcoidosis, amyloidosis, relapsing polychondritis, etc)

Infectious (eg, tuberculosis)

Tracheomalacia

more than 90% of reported patients with ISS are women, a hormonal influence has also been suggested. Estrogen, in particular, has been suggested as causative because it has been shown to play a role in fibrosis and keloid formation, but its role in ISS is yet to be elucidated.[6,9] Familial predisposition has not been established, although case reports of sisters and mothers and daughters developing ISS have been reported.[10] Some series have also found that body mass index is increased in women with ISS.[11]

ISS is defined by the endoscopic findings, which include a circumferential cicatricial stenosis that develops secondary to nonspecific inflammation, affects the proximal trachea and subglottic area, and is typically less than 2 cm in length.[2,12] Compared with patients with tracheal stenosis caused by other conditions, ISS tends to be shorter and located more proximally in the trachea.[3] Stenoses can be classified based on the Myer-Cotton classification, which equates endotracheal luminal size with degree of airway stenosis (**Table 1**).[13] Biopsy of the lesions shows fibrosis with or without acute inflammation.[14]

THERAPEUTIC OPTIONS: ENDOSCOPIC TREATMENT

Debate exists in the literature regarding the optimal treatment modality for patients with ISS. Generally, these patients are first managed endoscopically, both for diagnostic and therapeutic

Table 1
Myer-Cotton grade of airway obstruction

Grade	Obstruction (%)
I	50
II	51–75
III	>70 with any detectable lumen
IV	No detectable lumen

purposes. A first attempt at endoscopic treatment is often tried in the majority of patients with variable success.[6,15] Also, because the pathophysiology of ISS remains under debate, some investigators feel that endoscopic therapy is most appropriate because this process is slowly progressive and may recur in the future, even after definitive surgical resection.[16] Performing an endoscopic dilation of a subglottic stenosis can be therapeutic, yet can also aid in treatment planning, because it allows the surgeon to determine the length and severity of the stenosis. Advantages of endoscopic therapy include the lack of skin incision and the ability to discharge most patients on the day of the procedure. Also, endoscopic therapy is ideal for patients with ongoing active inflammation because these patients are not considered to be good surgical candidates until the active inflammation resolves.[3] Patients with long (>2 cm) or complex stenoses (with or without a malacic component) are at greater risk for failure of endoscopic therapy and thus considered to be better candidates for surgical management.[3,14]

Endoscopic Dilations

Dilation can be done using flexible bronchoscopy with balloon dilation, or rigid bronchoscopy with or without the use of gum-tipped bougie dilators. Performing dilation alone has been found to have a high rate of failure in patients with subglottic stenosis owing to all causes; thus, adjunctive modalities have been sought to improve these results.[17] Although patients with a diagnosis of ISS had a longer interval between dilations compared with other diagnoses, patients still required an average of 3 dilations, with some patients requiring up to 24 procedures.[18] Halmos and colleagues[19] found that patients with ISS required the most dilation bronchoscopies compared with other diagnoses. In contrast, another series found that, compared with patients who underwent dilation for stenosis caused by other etiologies, patients with ISS were found to have a significantly longer time between first and subsequent dilation.[20] Voice quality and production is a concern for many patients with ISS as because the stenosis is quite proximal and treatment can impact the vocal cord anatomy. The use of balloon dilation has been shown in a small series to improve dysphonia, which may be an advantage of endoscopic therapy compared with open surgical management.[21] Injections of the stricture with intralesional steroid or mitomycin have been described.[22] Although data are lacking for the efficacy of intralesional steroid injection to prevent stenosis recurrence, a small series found that the average interdilation interval was increased when steroids were used in addition to balloon dilation.[11]

Most interventions for ISS are done under general anesthesia, which comes with small risks and patients are often required to spend a night admitted to hospital for higher grade stenoses with the risk of airway edema after dilation. In an effort to improve on this technique, transcervical intralesional steroid injection performed as an outpatient procedure has been studied. This technique requires a minimum of 3 injections and has been shown to be safe in a small series, but requires further study to prove efficacy.[23]

Combined Modalities

In an effort to improve on the results of endoscopic dilation alone, this technique has been combined with other modalities, including laser incision, steroid injection, and mitomycin C injection. Laser incision is performed before dilatation in an effort to control the dilatation and prevent collateral tissue damage. However, this technique is not universally accepted therapy. In fact, we believe that the thermal injury from the laser is detrimental to healing and often generates more vigorous scar tissue formation that becomes transmural, making subsequent cricotracheal resection more challenging, and jeopardizing a good final result.

Mitomycin C is a chemotherapeutic agent that acts as a topical antifibrotic by cross-linking DNA and preventing the proliferation of fibroblasts by inducing apoptosis, thus decreasing the production of extracellular matrix proteins.[24] It is often used in combination with other modalities. Smith and Elstad[22] suggested that 2 applications result in a longer time before restenosis, but again, data are lacking regarding whether the addition of mitomycin C prevents restenosis.[6]

Some authors use multiple modalities in combination with low complication rates, such as laser radial incisions followed by balloon dilatation and injection of both mitomycin C and steroids.[3,25] Also, some groups have added postprocedure medical therapy with combinations of proton pump inhibitors, inhaled corticosteroids, and trimethoprim-sulfamethoxazole as part of the treatment algorithm and found encouraging results, but no controlled trials exist and more investigation is needed.[8,25] Nouraei and colleagues[26] report a success rate of 78% for combined modality endoscopic therapy, with an annual intervention rate of 1.07±0.79.

Most patients who have endoscopic treatment of ISS require multiple procedures (average, 2.4–4.2).[3,5,11,14] Parker and colleagues[3] found that the average time between procedures was 453 days. Although endoscopic therapy may be useful to delay surgical intervention, recurrence rates up to 70% have been reported.[8,11] Some patients may opt for repeated yearly dilations, however, to avoid surgical treatment.

THERAPEUTIC OPTIONS: SUBGLOTTIC TRACHEAL RESECTION AND SYNCHRONOUS CRICOID RESECTION

Cricotracheal resection provides definitive management for patients with subglottic stenosis, but it comes with unique technical challenges. Before the publication of Pearson's paper in 1975, options for the surgical management of subglottic stenosis were limited. For patients with intact nerves, this situation was not ideal. In addition to the issue of nerve preservation, resection of the entire cricoid resulted in loss of stability of the upper airway, thus affecting both speech and swallowing. Also, resections for subglottic stenosis affecting both the cricoid and trachea were often performed in 2 stages: the tracheal resection was performed by the thoracic surgeon, and the laryngeal resection was performed by the otolaryngologist. Owing to these difficulties, patients often were subjected to repeat dilatations, permanent tracheostomy, or, for malignancies affecting this location, total laryngectomy.[27] In 1975, Pearson published a report of 6 cases in which he performed single-stage subglottic tracheal resection with concomitant cricoid resection and reconstruction with preservation of the recurrent laryngeal nerves.

Preoperative Investigations

Preoperatively, all patients should be investigated using flexible bronchoscopy, as mentioned. This procedure is best done under general anesthesia with laryngeal mask airway (LMA) intubation. This technique allows the operator to have an excellent view of the larynx and well as the distal trachea and bronchial tree. One can perform balloon dilation through the LMA and then remove it to perform a rigid bronchoscopy for dilatation and measurement of the stricture length. It is also imperative to precisely define the anatomy using preoperative imaging. This is done with computed tomography scans of the neck with 3-dimensional tracheal reconstructions, which provide excellent surgically useful images from which the anatomy can be established with respect to location, length, and severity of obstruction (**Fig. 1**).

Patient Selection

There are no published guidelines to determine who would benefit most from cricotracheal

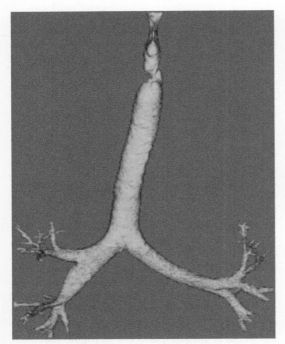

Fig. 1. Three-dimensional computed tomography tracheal reconstruction showing an area of stenosis.

resection. Factors that would suggest that patients who would do better with surgical management include those with multiple previous endoscopic interventions with recurrent or worsening stenosis, patient preference for a single procedure, long stenosis (>1-2 cm), and disorganized scar.[3,6] Often patients who present to a tertiary care center for cricotracheal resection have had at least 1 intervention elsewhere. Repeated unsuccessful interventions, especially if the dilations are difficult and tend to be traumatic to the airway, may worsen the stenosis by further contributing to acute and chronic inflammation. Most authors agree that any definitive surgical management should be delayed until any acute inflammation has subsided. As such, some patients may need endoscopic procedures as temporizing measures until the time of surgery.

Operative Technique

Patients are placed in the supine position with their neck slightly extended. This positioning is achieved using an inflatable bag placed behind the shoulders. To begin, after induction a LMA is placed, which allows bronchoscopy to be performed to confirm the operative plan. The LMA is kept in place until the time of tracheal transection, when the patient is switched to cross-field ventilation through a separate sterile circuit.

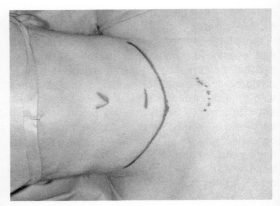

Fig. 2. Landmarking: cricoid cartilage superiorly, stenosis, skin incision, and sternal notch.

A collar incision is made (**Fig. 2**), the platysma is divided, and the strap muscles are separated (**Fig. 3**). The pretracheal plane is entered and dissected distally into the mediastinum and proximally to the larynx where the cricoid is cleared (**Fig. 4**). The trachea is mobilized laterally over a minimal distance spanning the area of stricture so as to minimize airway devascularization. Careful attention is paid to identify the recurrent laryngeal nerves on each side of the trachea (**Fig. 5**). The nerves run in the trachea–esophageal groove proximally to the posterolateral cricoid cartilage where they pass posterior to the cricothyroid joints (**Fig. 6**). In these operations for benign disease, the nerves need not be visualized because the dissection is carried out tightly on the edge of the trachea.

The cricoid cartilage is then dissected and resected anteriorly (**Figs. 7** and **8**). This is done by incising the airway in an oblique line from the inferior aspect of the thyroid cartilage superiorly to the lower edge of the cricoid plate

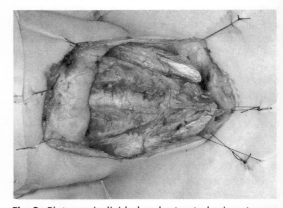

Fig. 3. Platysma is divided and retracted using stay sutures. The strap muscles are dissected.

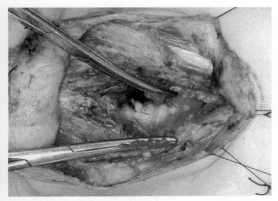

Fig. 4. The pretracheal plane is entered and the trachea is dissected.

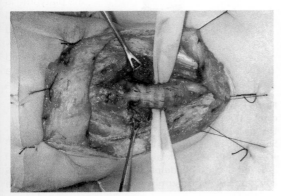

Fig. 5. The trachea is encircled using a Penrose drain.

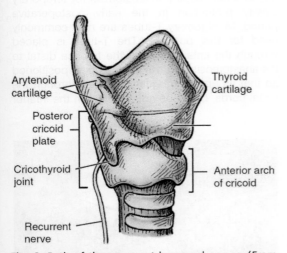

Arytenoid cartilage

Posterior cricoid plate

Cricothyroid joint

Recurrent nerve

Thyroid cartilage

Anterior arch of cricoid

Fig. 6. Path of the recurrent laryngeal nerves. (*From* Maddaus MA, Pearson FG. Subglottic resection: adults. In: Patterson GA, Cooper JD, Deslauriers J, et al, editors. Thoracic surgery. 3rd edition. Philadelphia: Churchill Livingstone; 2008. p. 354; with permission.)

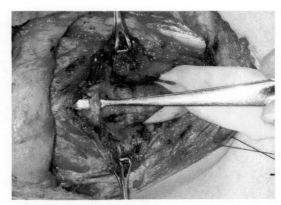

Fig. 7. The anterior cricoid arch is dissected free from surrounding tissue.

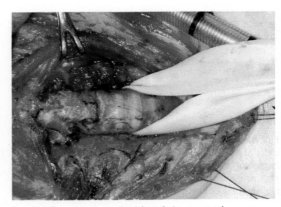

Fig. 8. The anterior cricoid arch is resected.

inferolaterally, below the area of the dissected nerves (**Fig. 9**). Thus, to preserve the recurrent laryngeal nerves, the posterior cricoid plate remains intact. The location of the distal transection is then identified and the trachea is divided at this level; stay sutures (3-0 polydioxanone suture) are placed at the junction of the cartilaginous and membranous airways distally (**Fig. 10**). The patient is then ventilated distally using cross-table ventilation, and the tissues overlying the posterior cricoid are dissected in the subperichondrial plane (**Fig. 11**). A Hall drill (#4 diamond burr tip) is used to flatten the luminal aspect of the posterior cricoid plate to provide a larger luminal aperture (**Fig. 12**). The posterior aspect of the cricoid plate is left intact, thus ensuring complete protection of the recurrent laryngeal nerves. This resection of the posterior aspect of the cricoid can be continued almost until the vocal cords. The normal proximal mucosa at the inferior border of the thyroid cartilage is then divided. The line of mucosal division is proximal to the line of airway transection, and within 1 cm of the vocal cords (**Fig. 13**).

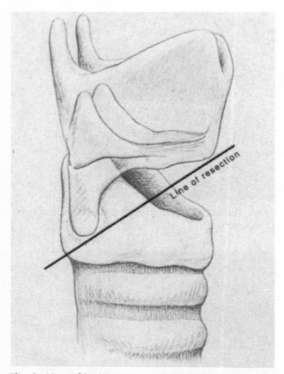

Fig. 9. Line of incision across the cricoid. (*From* Maddaus MA, Pearson FG. Subglottic resection: adults. In: Patterson GA, Cooper JD, Deslauriers J, et al, editors. Thoracic surgery. 3rd edition. Philadelphia: Churchill Livingstone; 2008. p. 354; with permission.)

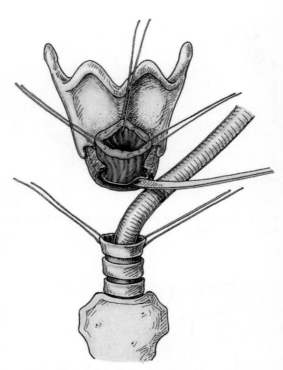

Fig. 11. The cricoid is dissected in the subperichondrial plane, and cross-table ventilation is used into the distal trachea. (*From* Maddaus MA, Pearson FG. Subglottic resection: adults. In: Patterson GA, Cooper JD, Deslauriers J, et al, editors. Thoracic surgery. 3rd edition. Philadelphia: Churchill Livingstone; 2008. p. 354; with permission.)

The proximal and distal ends of the airway are brought together to test the tension on the anastomosis. The inflatable bag behind the shoulders is deflated to facilitate this check, and slight neck flexion may also be used. The anastomosis is performed using running 4-0 polydioxanone suture for the posterior membranous wall (**Fig. 14**). Interrupted 4-0 or 3-0 polydioxanone suture is used to perform the anastomosis of the cartilaginous wall anteriorly (**Fig. 15**).

Whereas Pearson's original article described the use of small metal tracheostomies for temporary airway protection in the early postoperative period, Montgomery T-tubes are now commonly used for this purpose. The T-tube is placed through the anterior wall of the trachea distal to the anastomosis (**Fig. 16**). The T-tube is positioned so that its upper limb just protrudes through the vocal cords, but does not impinge on the inferior

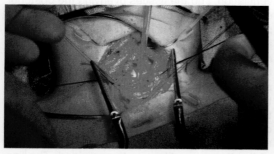

Fig. 10. The trachea is transected at the distal margin and the specimen is removed. Stay sutures are placed on the junction of the cartilage and membranous wall of the trachea distally.

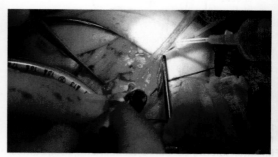

Fig. 12. The posterior lamina of the cricoid is drilled to permit greater proximal resection.

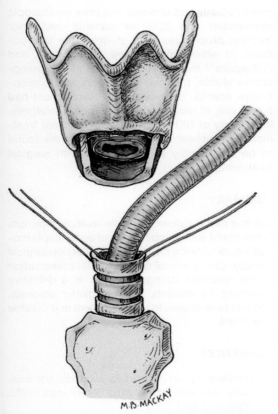

Fig. 13. The dissection is complete. (*From* Maddaus MA, Pearson FG. Subglottic resection: adults. In: Patterson GA, Cooper JD, Deslauriers J, et al, editors. Thoracic surgery. 3rd edition. Philadelphia: Churchill Livingstone; 2008. p. 354; with permission.)

surface of the epiglottis. The positioning of the T-tube is facilitated by visualization with the flexible fiberoptic bronchoscope through the LMA with the patient's neck in the neutral position as the operating surgeons are inserting the tube. The strap muscles and platysma are

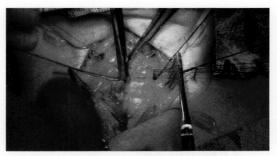

Fig. 15. The anterior portion of the anastomosis is performed using interrupted 4-0 polydioxanone suture sutures.

reapproximated and the subcutaneous tissue is sutured (**Fig. 17**). The T-tube is brought out through the skin usually though a separate appropriately sited skin incision and a 10 flat Jackson-Pratt drain is placed below the muscle layers adjacent to the anastomosis and into the lowest reach of dissection of the pretracheal plane into the mediastinum. The skin is closed with staples. A large skin suture is places from the chin to the manubrium (the Pearson chin stitch) to keep the neck in neutral position and remind the patient to avoid extreme extension, which pulls on the tracheal anastomosis. This stitch is kept in place for 5 days postoperatively (**Fig. 18**).

CLINICAL OUTCOMES OF CRICOTRACHEAL RESECTION

In 1973, Pearson reported his first 28 patients who underwent cricoid resection with thyrotracheal anastomosis. Of these 28 patients, preservation of the recurrent laryngeal nerves was attempted in 21 and successful in 20. Two patients experienced a partial restenosis, leaving 26 patients with no evidence of restenosis, with the 5- to 10-year follow-up reported on 19 of the 28 patients.[28] D'Andrilli and colleagues[29] reported

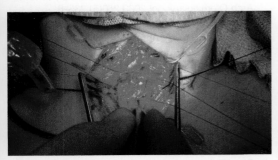

Fig. 14. The posterior membranous wall anastomosis is performed using running 4-0 polydioxanone suture sutures.

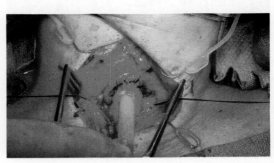

Fig. 16. The anastomosis is complete and the T-tube is in place.

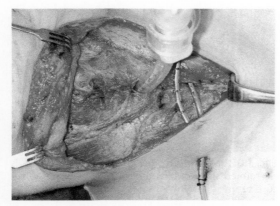

Fig. 17. The strap muscles are reapproximated around the T-tube.

on their experience with Pearson's technique. For all-comers, 90.8 of patients had excellent or good results, with minor complications in only 4 patients. This group modified the original technique by replacing the T-tube that Pearson described with an uncuffed nasotracheal tube that is removed at 24 hours after bronchoscopy to confirm patency of the anastomosis. Morcillo and colleagues[30] reported on 60 patients who had tracheal resection for ISS using a variety of techniques, and found that 17 of the 18 patients (94%) who had resection using the Pearson technique had excellent results.

Using a similar technique, Grillo and associates[15] reported on 73 patients who underwent surgical resection of ISS and found that 90% of patients had good or excellent results. More than 60% of patients had change in their voice after this technique, with most of the issues affecting voice projection and singing.[15] The same group updated their results in 2015 and reported improved results with 96% of patients experiencing a good or excellent result; 70% of

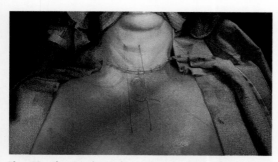

Fig. 18. The T-tube is brought out through the skin and the incision is closed with staples. One small drain is left in place. The chin is sutured to the anterior chest wall.

these patients had undergone a prior endoscopic intervention and 22% of patients had prior tracheal procedures.[31] In studying the 263 patients of which only 2 were male, Wang and colleagues[31] found that patients who had preoperative stents, previous mitomycin use, postoperative edema, and vocal cord involvement had a high risk of recurrent stenosis postoperatively. In a survey of 160 patients who underwent treatment for tracheal stenosis, patients were found to be significantly more satisfied with surgical treatment.[32]

SUMMARY

ISS is a rare diagnosis. Despite multiple attempts at treatment with combinations of endoscopic modalities, recurrence rates are high after nonsurgical therapy. Cricotracheal resection with preservation of the recurrent laryngeal nerves is a definitive treatment for patients with subglottic stenosis, and has been shown to have excellent and durable outcomes.

REFERENCES

1. Brandenburg JH. Idiopathic subglottic stenosis. Trans Am Acad Ophthalmol Otolaryngol 1972; 76(5):1402–6.
2. Pearson FG. Idiopathic laryngotracheal stenosis. J Thorac Cardiovasc Surg 2004;127(1):10–1.
3. Parker NP, Bandyopadhyay D, Misono S, et al. Endoscopic cold incision, balloon dilation, mitomycin C application, and steroid injection for adult laryngotracheal stenosis. Laryngoscope 2013; 123(1):220–5.
4. Ashiku SK, Kuzucu A, Grillo HC, et al. Idiopathic laryngotracheal stenosis: effective definitive treatment with laryngotracheal resection. J Thorac Cardiovasc Surg 2004;127(1):99–107.
5. Giudice M, Piazza C, Foccoli P, et al. Idiopathic subglottic stenosis: management by endoscopic and open-neck surgery in a series of 30 patients. Eur Arch Otorhinolaryngol 2003;260(5):235–8.
6. Valdez TA, Shapshay SM. Idiopathic subglottic stenosis revisited. Ann Otol Rhinol Laryngol 2002; 111(8):690–5.
7. Terra RM, de Medeiros IL, Minamoto H, et al. Idiopathic tracheal stenosis: successful outcome with antigastroesophageal reflux disease therapy. Ann Thorac Surg 2008;85(4):1438–9.
8. Maldonado F, Loiselle A, Depew ZS, et al. Idiopathic subglottic stenosis: an evolving therapeutic algorithm. Laryngoscope 2014;124(2):498–503.
9. Chau D, Mancoll JS, Lee S, et al. Tamoxifen downregulates TGF-beta production in keloid fibroblasts. Ann Plast Surg 1998;40(5):490–3.

10. Dumoulin E, Stather DR, Gelfand G, et al. Idiopathic subglottic stenosis: a familial predisposition. Ann Thorac Surg 2013;95(3):1084–6.

11. Shabani S, Hoffman MR, Brand WT, et al. Endoscopic management of idiopathic subglottic stenosis. Ann Otol Rhinol Laryngol 2017;126(2):96–102.

12. Liberman M, Mathisen DJ. Treatment of idiopathic laryngotracheal stenosis. Semin Thorac Cardiovasc Surg 2009;21(3):278–83.

13. Myer CM, O'Connor DM, Cotton RT. Proposed grading system for subglottic stenosis based on endotracheal tube sizes. Ann Otol Rhinol Laryngol 1994;103(4 Pt 1):319–23.

14. Park SS, Streitz JM, Rebeiz EE, et al. Idiopathic subglottic stenosis. Arch Otolaryngol Head Neck Surg 1995;121(8):894–7.

15. Grillo HC, Mathisen DJ, Ashiku SK, et al. Successful treatment of idiopathic laryngotracheal stenosis by resection and primary anastomosis. Ann Otol Rhinol Laryngol 2003;112(9 Pt 1):798–800.

16. Dedo HH, Catten MD. Idiopathic progressive subglottic stenosis: findings and treatment in 52 patients. Ann Otol Rhinol Laryngol 2001;110(4): 305–11.

17. Simpson GT, Strong MS, Healy GB, et al. Predictive factors of success or failure in the endoscopic management of laryngeal and tracheal stenosis. Ann Otol Rhinol Laryngol 1982;91(4 Pt 1):384–8.

18. Kocdor P, Siegel ER, Suen JY, et al. Comorbidities and factors associated with endoscopic surgical outcomes in adult laryngotracheal stenosis. Eur Arch Otorhinolaryngol 2016;273(2):419–24.

19. Halmos GB, Schuiringa FS, Pálinkó D, et al. Finding balance between minimally invasive surgery and laryngotracheal resection in the management of adult laryngotracheal stenosis. Eur Arch Otorhinolaryngol 2014;271(7):1967–71.

20. Gadkaree SK, Pandian V, Best S, et al. Laryngotracheal stenosis: risk factors for tracheostomy dependence and dilation interval. Otolaryngol Head Neck Surg 2017;156(2):321–8.

21. Hoffman MR, Brand WT, Dailey SH. Effects of balloon dilation for idiopathic laryngotracheal stenosis on voice production. Ann Otol Rhinol Laryngol 2016;125(1):12–9.

22. Smith ME, Elstad M. Mitomycin C and the endoscopic treatment of laryngotracheal stenosis: are two applications better than one? Laryngoscope 2009;119(2):272–83.

23. Hoffman MR, Coughlin AR, Dailey SH. Serial office-based steroid injections for treatment of idiopathic subglottic stenosis. Laryngoscope 2017;127(11): 2475–81.

24. Gray SD, Tritle N, Li W. The effect of mitomycin on extracellular matrix proteins in a rat wound model. Laryngoscope 2003;113(2):237–42.

25. Gouveris H, Karaiskaki N, Koutsimpelas D, et al. Treatment for adult idiopathic and Wegener-associated subglottic stenosis. Eur Arch Otorhinolaryngol 2013;270(3):989–93.

26. Nouraei SA, Sandhu GS. Outcome of a multimodality approach to the management of idiopathic subglottic stenosis. Laryngoscope 2013;123(10): 2474–84.

27. Pearson FG, Cooper JD, Nelems JM, et al. Primary tracheal anastomosis after resection of the cricoid cartilage with preservation of recurrent laryngeal nerves. J Thorac Cardiovasc Surg 1975;70(5): 806–16.

28. Pearson FG, Brito-Filomeno L, Cooper JD. Experience with partial cricoid resection and thyrotracheal anastomosis. Ann Otol Rhinol Laryngol 1986;95(6 Pt 1):582–5.

29. D'Andrilli A, Maurizi G, Andreetti C, et al. Long-term results of laryngotracheal resection for benign stenosis from a series of 109 consecutive patients. Eur J Cardiothorac Surg 2016;50(1):105–9.

30. Morcillo A, Wins R, Gómez-Caro A, et al. Single-staged laryngotracheal reconstruction for idiopathic tracheal stenosis. Ann Thorac Surg 2013; 95(2):433–9 [discussion: 9].

31. Wang H, Wright CD, Wain JC, et al. Idiopathic subglottic stenosis: factors affecting outcome after single-stage repair. Ann Thorac Surg 2015;100(5): 1804–11.

32. Gnagi SH, Howard BE, Anderson C, et al. Idiopathic subglottic and tracheal stenosis: a survey of the patient experience. Ann Otol Rhinol Laryngol 2015; 124(9):734–9.

Partial Cricotracheal Resection and Extended Cricotracheal Resection for Pediatric Laryngotracheal Stenosis

Philippe Monnier, MD*

KEYWORDS

- Pediatric • Laryngotracheal stenosis • Subglottic stenosis • Cricotracheal resection
- Laryngotracheal reconstruction • Stents • Infants • Children

KEY POINTS

- Train yourself adequately in laryngotracheal surgery and upper airway endoscopy before addressing the challenging surgery of pediatric laryngotracheal stenosis (LTS).
- Remember that inappropriate initial management of LTS can lead to permanent intractable sequelae and that the patients' best chance lies in the first operation.
- Perform a thorough preoperative assessment of the patients' medical condition and of the stenosis to choose the best surgical option and timing.
- Master all types of surgical techniques starting from appropriate use of the carbon-dioxide laser for minor intrinsic stenoses to laryngotracheal reconstruction with cartilage expansion, partial cricotracheal resection, and extended-cricotracheal resection for the more severe grades of LTS.

INTRODUCTION

Pediatric airway surgery encompasses a wide array of endoscopic and open procedures developed over the last decades to treat a variety of pathologic conditions of the larynx and trachea in infants and children. These conditions include congenital anomalies (laryngomalacia, bilateral vocal fold paralysis, subglottic stenosis, vocal fold webbing, laryngeal atresia, saccular cysts, laryngoceles, laryngotracheoesophageal clefts)[1,2] and acquired conditions resulting from prolonged intubation,[3] external and internal trauma, and rare neoplasias.

It is beyond the scope of this short essay to describe all of the endoscopic and surgical interventions that are needed to address such a variety of different pathologies. This article focuses instead on the yield of partial cricotracheal resection (PCTR) and extended-PCTR (E-PCTR) used for the management of congenital and acquired laryngotracheal stenosis (LTS) in infants and children.

Acquired LTS in the pediatric age group differs significantly from adult LTS for the following reasons:

1. Subglottic stenosis (SGS) is more often associated with glottic involvement, mainly

Disclosure Statement: The author will hold a financial relationship with the stent manufacturer, if the LT-Mold makes it to the market (which is not yet the case).
Otolaryngology, Head and Neck Surgery Department, University Hospital CHUV, Rue du Bugnon 46, Lausanne CH 1011, Switzerland
* Boulevard de la Forêt 36, Pully CH 1009, Switzerland.
E-mail address: monnier.phido@gmail.com

posterior glottic stenosis (PGS), vocal fold synechia, or transglottic stenosis (28 of 141 = 33% of the cases in the authors' series of patients). This situation usually requires an interarytenoid expansion with a posterior costal cartilage graft (PCCG) combined with a subglottic resection, the so-called E-PCTR. But in many cases, PGS is not combined with SGS or only with a minor degree of SGS, so laryngotracheal reconstruction (LTR) with PCCG is usually sufficient to restore an adequate airway.[4]

2. The size of the subglottis is much smaller in infants and children than in adults. This smaller size implies a more challenging postextubation period in the pediatric intensive care unit (PICU) after single-stage PCTR and a perfect mucosal approximation at the anastomotic site during the surgery to avoid granulation tissue formation and restenosis.[5]

3. Finally, pulmonary and neurologic sequelae from prematurity or congenital (cardiac, esophageal or maxillofacial) anomalies often add to the therapeutic challenge.

PREOPERATIVE WORKUP

A thorough endoscopic evaluation usually provides all of the information needed for careful planning of the surgery.[6]

If precise description and measurements of the LTS are obtained from the endoscopy, then radiographs add little to the preoperative workup, because laryngeal cartilages show poorly on computed tomography (CT)-scan images in infants and children. However, 3-dimensional CT-scan or MRI reconstructions are useful for assessing intrathoracic airway narrowing secondary to congenital cardiovascular anomalies or rare tumors.[7]

Endoscopic Assessment

- Transnasal bronchofiberscopy under spontaneous respiration is performed to assess vocal fold (VF) mobility and all potential sites of extralaryngeal obstruction (naso-oropharynx, tracheostoma, distal trachea, and bronchi).[8]
- Rigid direct laryngotracheoscopy with a bare 0° telescope is used to precisely assess the location, extent, and size of the SGS; the exact location of the tracheostoma with respect to the stenosis; and the number of residual normal tracheal rings situated below the tracheostoma.
- Suspended microlaryngoscopy is implemented in case of VF immobility to differentiate neurogenic VF paralysis from PGS, potentially with cicatricial cricoarytenoid joint fixation.
- In the pediatric community, the Meyer-Cotton airway grading system is routinely used as a predictor of success or failure after LTR used for the cure of SGS.[9] But more recently, implementation of glottic involvement and patients' comorbidities to the degree of SGS has shown to be the best predictors of outcome following PCTR and E-PCTR because the diseased airway segment is fully resected during the surgery[10] (**Table 1**).
- Finally, a bacteriologic aspirate of the trachea is systematically taken to look for resistant bacteria that require proper treatment before the surgery. Failure to do so may ruin the final result of PCTR, E-PCTR, or LTR.

Patients' General Condition

- A full medical history of the cause of the SGS, including the cause for long-term intubation, should be obtained.[11]

Table 1
Modified Myer-Cotton airway grading system

Myer-Cotton Grade	Isolated SGS (a)	Isolated SGS + Comorbidities (b)	SGS + Glottic Involvement (c)	SGS + Glottic Involvement + Comorbidities (d)
I	0%–50%	SGS Ia	SGS Ib	SGS Ic	SGS Id
II	51%–70%	SGS IIa	SGS IIb	SGS IIc	SGS IId
III	71%–99%	SGS IIIa	SGS IIIb	SGS IIIc	SGS IIId
IV	No lumen	SGS IVa	SGS IVb	SGS IVc	SGS IVd

From Monnier P. Preoperative assessment, indications for surgery and parental counselling. In: Monnier P, editor. Pediatric airway surgery. Berlin: Springer Verlag; 2011. p. 234; with permission.

- Cardiopulmonary function should be assessed in children with a history of prematurity or congenital anomalies.
- Full evaluation of patients' congenital anomalies or comorbidities should include neurologic, cardiac, and pulmonary examinations; swallowing function tests; gastroesophageal reflux measurements; and maxillofacial evaluation, when deemed necessary.

INDICATIONS FOR LARYNGOTRACHEAL RECONSTRUCTION, PARTIAL CRICOTRACHEAL RESECTION, EXTENDED PARTIAL CRICOTRACHEAL RESECTION, AND AIRWAY STENTING

Primary endoscopic treatment of thin, weblike SGS may still be used in select cases; but if the result of carbon-dioxide laser/dilatation leads to a recurrence of the stenosis to its initial grade, then any further endoscopic treatment is strictly contraindicated. Open surgery should be considered instead.[12]

Laryngotracheal Reconstruction

- In the otolaryngology community, single- or double-stage LTR is still used for treating isolated grade I (<50%), grade II (51%–70%), and some mild grade III (up to 80% airway obstruction) SGS. However, troublesome wound healing with exposed cartilage, granulation tissue formation, and restenosis increases with the severity of the SGS.
- LTR remains the sole option for treating PGS (isolated or combined with a minor degree of

SGS), as it requires an expansion of the posterior laryngeal commissure with a costal cartilage graft in most, if not all, pediatric cases.

Partial Cricotracheal Resection and Extended Partial Cricotracheal Resection

- Single-stage PCTR is used for treating isolated grade II (51%–70%), grade III (71%–99% airway obstruction), and grade IV (no detectable lumen) SGS in an otherwise healthy infant or child (**Fig. 1**).
- Double-stage PCTR is preferred for the same abovementioned indications in children with compromised neurologic or cardiopulmonary functions, with swallowing problems, mental disabilities, or multiple congenital anomalies.
- Double-stage E-PCTR with stenting is used for treating grade III and IV SGSs associated with cicatricial or congenital glottic involvement (acquired SGS + PGS or VF synechia; congenital SGS + extensive VF webbing or laryngeal atresia) (**Fig. 2**).

Airway stenting

Stents should not be used in the airway unless there is no other solution to resolve the problem. Although they provide support to airway reconstructions, stents can act as foreign bodies and induce mucosal injuries, ulcerations, granulation tissue formation, and subsequent restenosis.

At the level of the larynx, stents are necessary when the SGS involves the glottis (PGS or VF synechia) and/or supraglottis (transglottic stenosis). Unfortunately, none of the stents

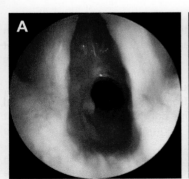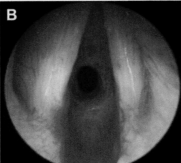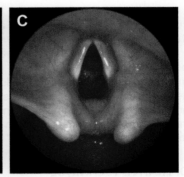

Fig. 1. Isolated SGS. (*A*) Grade II SGS. (*B*) Grade III SGS. (*C*) Grade IV SGS. (*From* [*B*] Monnier P. Endoscopic assessment of the compromised paediatric airway. In: Pediatric airway surgery. Berlin: Springer Verlag; 2011. p. 84; with permission; and [*C*] Monnier P. Endoscopic assessment of the compromised paediatric airway. In: Monnier P, editor. Pediatric airway surgery. Berlin: Springer Verlag; 2011. p. 92; with permission.)

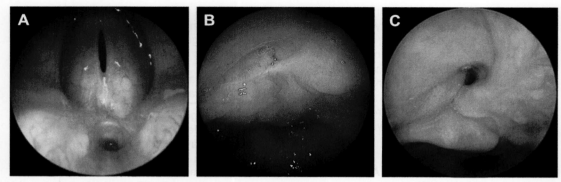

Fig. 2. Complex laryngotracheal stenosis. (*A*) Glotto-SGS. (*B*) Transglottic stenosis. (*C*) Distorted larynx resulting from failed LTR. (*From* [*A*] Monnier P. Acquired post-intubation and tracheostomy-related stenoses. In: Pediatric airway surgery. Berlin: Springer Verlag; 2011. p. 188; with permission. [*B*] Monnier P. Endoscopic assessment of the compromised paediatric airway. In: Pediatric airway surgery. Berlin: Springer Verlag; 2011. p. 92; with permission. [*C*] Monnier P. Laryngotracheoplasty and laryngotracheal reconstruction. In: Monnier P, editor. Pediatric airway surgery. Berlin: Springer Verlag; 2011. p. 265; with permission.)

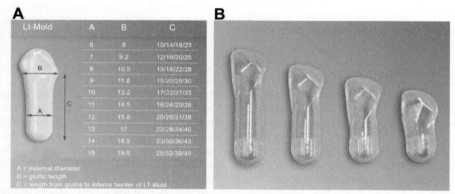

Fig. 3. LT-Mold. (*A*) The prosthesis exists in 10 different sizes (6–15 mm in outer diameter) for use in infants, children, and adults. (*B*) Per size, the prosthesis exists in 4 different lengths to accommodate different positions of the tracheostomy site. (*From* [*A*] Monnier P. Applied surgical anatomy of the larynx and trachea. In: Pediatric airway surgery. Berlin: Springer Verlag; 2011. p. 24; with permission; and [*B*] Monnier P. Applied surgical anatomy of the larynx and trachea. In: Monnier P, editor. Pediatric airway surgery. Berlin: Springer Verlag; 2011. p. 25; with permission.)

currently available on the market are suitable for the larynx.

To overcome this problem, the LT-Mold has been designed more recently.[13] It conforms to the inner contours of a fully abducted larynx, a key feature when considering restoration of the anterior laryngeal commissure and of a normal interarytenoid distance, after an E-PCTR performed for glotto-SGS (**Fig. 3**).

OPERATIVE TECHNIQUE
Partial Cricotracheal Resection

In infants and children, the surgery is performed in a similar fashion as in the adult population[14,15]:

- The dissection of the trachea is carried out in close contact with the tracheal rings, without identifying the recurrent laryngeal nerves (RLNs).
- The vascular supply to the trachea, coming from the tracheoesophageal grooves, is carefully preserved, except over the segment that needs to be resected.
- The upper limit of the tracheal dissection does not extend more cranially than the lower edge of the cricoid ring to avoid injury to the RLNs.
- The following steps of the surgery are depicted in **Figs. 4–7**.

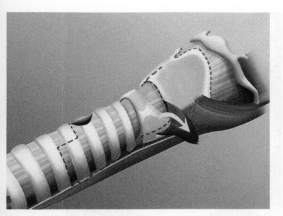

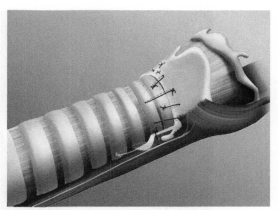

Fig. 4. Pediatric PCTR: resection lines. Both cricothyroid muscles are sharply dissected off the anterior arch of the cricoid ring and reflected laterally over the cricothyroid joints, thus, protecting the RLNs that run just posterior to them. On the diagram, the RLN is shown for anatomic purposes only. The superior resection line is made at the inferior margin of the thyroid cartilage and passes laterally just in front of both cricothyroid joints. The inferior resection line is carried out one ring below the first normal tracheal ring (usually just below the tracheostoma in single-stage PCTR) to harvest an anterior pedicled wedge of cartilage that will be used to enlarge the subglottic lumen. (*From* Monnier P. Partial cricotracheal resection. In: Monnier P, editor. Pediatric airway surgery. Berlin: Springer Verlag; 2011. p. 288; with permission.)

Fig. 6. Pediatric PCTR: Anastomosis. Except for the most posterolateral sutures, which are placed between the trachea and the cricoid plate, all lateral and anterior stitches are passed between the tracheal rings and the thyroid cartilage. The triangular defect resulting from the inferior midline thyrotomy is filled in with the cartilaginous wedge pedicled to the tracheal ring used for the anastomosis. (*From* Monnier P. Partial cricotracheal resection. In: Monnier P, editor. Pediatric airway surgery. Berlin: Springer Verlag; 2011. p. 291; with permission.)

Extended Partial Cricotracheal Resection

The basic principles of E-PCTR are identical to that of PCTR, but 2 additional steps are taken[16] (**Figs. 8–11**).

SPECIFIC RECOMMENDATIONS
Primary Location of the Tracheostoma

In case of fresh, incipient SGS, the tracheostoma should be placed either between the cricoid and first tracheal ring or as low as possible in the neck (sixth or seventh tracheal ring in children whereby the larynx lies in a very rostral position) (**Fig. 12**). In the former situation, a single-stage PCTR with limited (2–3 rings) tracheal resection is easily performed, should a mature cicatricial stenosis develop. In the latter situation, vascu-

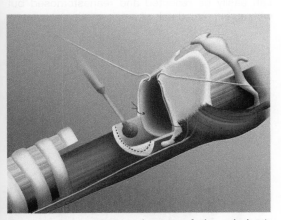

Fig. 5. Pediatric PCTR: reshaping of the subglottic space. After resection of the anterior arch of the cricoid, the fibrous tissue constituting the posterior aspect of the stenosis is fully resected. The transverse section of the posterior subglottic mucosa is made just a few millimeters below the level of the vocal folds. The denuded cricoid plate is then flattened with a diamond burr, which facilitates proper adaptation of the tracheal stump to the subglottis. In infants and children, the subglottis must be enlarged to match the size of the tracheal stump. This enlargement is obtained by performing an inferior midline incision of the thyroid cartilage, staying just below

the anterior laryngeal commissure to preserve a good voice. Because the thyroid cartilage is soft and pliable in children, the subglottic circumference can be spread by a few millimeters, which increases the cross-sectional area of the subglottis significantly. An additional measure is to fix the lateral subglottic mucosa with 5.0 polyglactin 910 (Vicryl, Ethicon Inc, Somerville, NJ) or PDS sutures to the inferior margin of the thyroid cartilage to open the lumen laterally. (*From* Monnier P. Partial cricotracheal resection. In: Monnier P, editor. Pediatric airway surgery. Berlin: Springer Verlag; 2011. p. 289; with permission.)

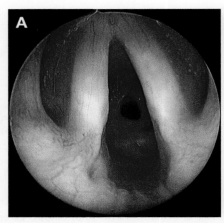 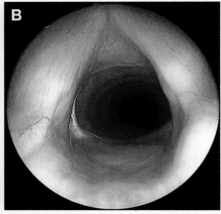

Fig. 7. Single-stage PCTR for isolated grade III SGS. (*A*) Preoperative view. (*B*) Postoperative view 2 years after surgery. (*From* Monnier P. Partial cricotracheal resection. In: Pediatric airway surgery. Berlin: Springer Verlag; 2011. p. 292; with permission.)

larity of the tracheal rings situated above the tracheostoma is well preserved and allows for a short (cricoid resection only) double-stage PCTR without any risk of anastomotic dehiscence.

Knowing that the risk of anastomotic dehiscence is proportional to the length of tracheal resection and devascularization, correct placement of the tracheostoma for incipient SGS should be known by all surgeons. This ability would significantly improve the outcome of LTS surgery.

Extensive airway resection

Permissible length of airway resection varies individually with patients' complexion and prior surgery. In infants and children, 50% of the trachea can easily be resected and reanastomosed but with an increased risk of anastomotic dehiscence

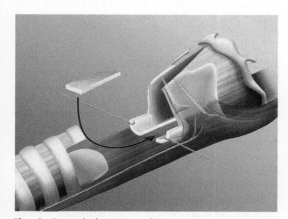

Fig. 8. Extended PCTR: Additional steps to simple PCTR. A full laryngofissure is carried out to gain access to the cricoid plate that is divided in the midline to spread the narrowed interarytenoid space, site of the PGS. A costal cartilage graft is interposed between the divided cricoid laminae, and a pedicled flap of membranous trachea is obtained by removing 2 additional rings of the tracheal stump distally. This procedure also allows the delineation of the anterior cartilaginous wedge that will be used to fill in the triangular defect resulting from the inferior midline thyrotomy. (*From* Monnier P. Partial cricotracheal resection. In: Monnier P, editor. Pediatric airway surgery. Berlin: Springer Verlag; 2011. p. 294; with permission.)

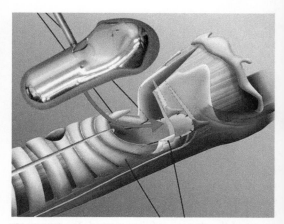

Fig. 9. Extended PCTR: Creating a fully mucosalized airway. The trachea is advanced cranially, and its membranous portion is sutured to the widened interarytenoid mucosa. Thus, a fully mucosalized airway is recreated. A gauge is used to select the proper size LT-Mold that will stabilize the reconstruction until full mucosal healing is obtained. (*From* Monnier P. Partial cricotracheal resection. In: Monnier P, editor. Pediatric airway surgery. Berlin: Springer Verlag; 2011. p. 295; with permission.)

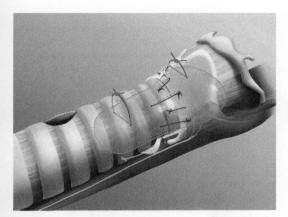

Fig. 10. Extended PCTR: Anastomosis. After tying the posterolateral stitches, the silicone LT-Mold prosthesis is introduced into the airway. Care is taken to reposition the anterior laryngeal commissure precisely and to fix the LT-Mold at this level with a resorbable 5.0 Vicryl suture to avoid granulation tissue formation. The cranial part of the laryngofissure is then closed with interrupted Vicryl sutures, and the LT-Mold is securely fixed to the airway by two 3.0 polypropylene (Prolene, Ethicon, Inc, Somerville, NJ) sutures (*in red on the diagram*). The lateral and anterior anastomosis is completed as in conventional PCTR with the pedicled wedge of tracheal cartilage filling in the triangular defect of the inferior midline thyrotomy. (*From* Monnier P. Partial cricotracheal resection. In: Monnier P, editor. Pediatric airway surgery. Berlin: Springer Verlag; 2011. p. 296; with permission.)

(3.5% for resection of <5 rings vs 12.5% for resection of 6–8 rings in the authors' own series of 141 patients).

Recapture of tracheal length

In the pediatric age group, the infrahyoid release is preferred because the thyroid cartilage is partially concealed behind the hyoid bone (**Fig. 13**).

In the authors' cohort of 141 pediatric patients who underwent PCTR or E-PCTR, a laryngeal release maneuver was done in 28 (20%) patients; but a partial anterior release (section of the thyrohyoid membrane only) was routinely performed in almost all cases.

Hilar and pericardial releases are not necessary even for long tracheal resections, because mobilization of the tracheal stump is much easier in children than in adults.

POSTOPERATIVE CARE

- Antibiotics based on culture sensitivities and antireflux medication are given until a fully mucosalized subglottis is obtained after PCTR, E-PCTR, or LTR.
- Infants and children are kept intubated, sedated, or paralyzed in the PICU after single-stage PCTR and double-stage E-PCTR to minimize the risk of anastomotic dehiscence.
- Extubation is attempted at day 5 or 7 after single-stage PCTR.
- After extubation, continuous positive airway pressure is delivered through a face mask to counteract the Bernoulli effect at the level of the swollen (due to the proximity of the anastomosis) VFs.
- Control endoscopies are performed before extubation and to any reintubation, but

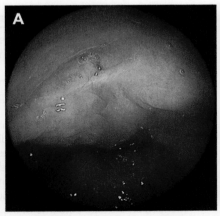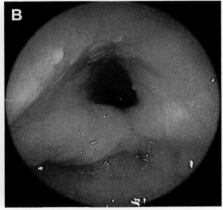

Fig. 11. Extended PCTR for transglottic stenosis. (*A*) Preoperative view: The vocal folds are fused together, and a posterior supraglottic band of scar tissue is conspicuous. (*B*) Postoperative view: Patent glotto-subglottic airway, albeit with a slightly distorted interarytenoid space. (*From* Monnier P. Partial cricotracheal resection. In: Monnier P, editor. Pediatric airway surgery. Berlin: Springer Verlag; 2011. p. 299; with permission.)

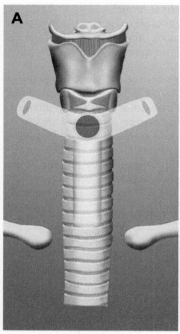
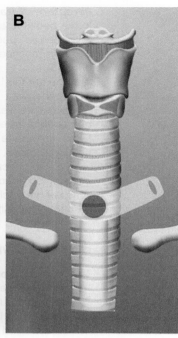

Fig. 12. Correct placement of tracheotomy for impending SGS. (*A*) Tracheostoma situated immediately below the cricoid ring to maximally preserve the normal trachea. (*B*) Tracheostoma situated at the sixth to seventh tracheal rings to spare a sufficient length of well-vascularized, normal trachea between the SGS and the tracheostomy. (*From* Monnier P. Acquired post-intubation and tracheostomy-related stenoses. In: Monnier P, editor. Pediatric airway surgery. Berlin: Springer Verlag; 2011. p. 195; with permission.)

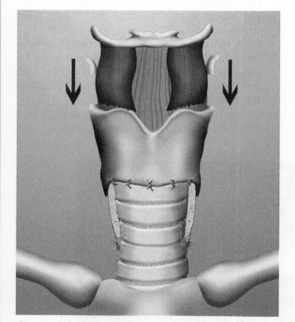

Fig. 13. Infrahyoid laryngeal release maneuver. The sternohyoid and thyrohyoid muscles are divided at their insertion level on the thyroid cartilage. The thyrohyoid membrane is sectioned along the upper rim of the thyroid cartilage, reaching the superior cornua of the thyroid cartilage, which are sectioned bilaterally using Mayo scissors. A 1.5- to 2.0-cm-long release is obtained.

routinely at 3 weeks and 3 months postoperatively.
- Dilatation of the anastomotic site is never performed before the sixth postoperative week, in case of a suboptimal result.

COMPLICATIONS

Complications usually result from insufficient preoperative assessment and/or failure of the surgical technique.

Insufficient Preoperative Assessment

- Inadequate evaluation of the stenosis, imprecise assessment of VF function, missed concomitant airway lesions, and failure to obtain a bacteriologic aspirate of the trachea can all lead to complications and a poor result of the surgery.
- Failure to identify congenital anomalies, lung disease caused by prematurity, cardiovascular problems, airway infection, gastroesophageal reflux, eosinophilic esophagitis, feeding difficulties and aspiration, neurologic impairment and mental disability has deleterious consequences on the final outcome of the surgery.

A check list of the patients' assessment (endoscopy and comorbidities) should routinely be used to avoid missing any important information that can have a strong negative impact on the final outcome of the surgery.[6]

Failure of the Surgical Technique

Anastomotic dehiscence can result from excessive anastomotic tension, undue tracheal devascularization, inappropriate anastomotic technique, or superinfection.

These complications can be avoided by the following measures:

- Extensive intrathoracic mobilization of the trachea and full infrahyoid laryngeal release
- Preservation of all vascular supply to the trachea, except over the resected segment
- Passing all anastomotic stitches in the submucosal plane to preserve the vascular supply to the anastomosis
- Giving antibiotics based on culture sensitivities for airway colonization with resistant bacteria

Recurrent stenosis results from a slow, progressive anastomotic dehiscence that leads to granulation tissue formation and cicatricial contraction. As for anastomotic dehiscence, this complication increases with the length of airway that needs to be resected.

RLN injury can be avoided by not identifying the RLNs but dissecting the trachea short of the tracheal rings, limiting cranial dissection of the trachea to the level of the inferior margin of the cricoid plate, and protecting the RLNs by reflecting both cricothyroid muscles laterally over the cricothyroid joints (see **Fig. 4**). Permanent RLN injury only occurred in 1 of 141 (0.7%) patients of the author' series, in a difficult revision surgery with obscured anatomy at the level of the cricoid.

RESULTS

Evaluation of outcomes following pediatric subglottic resection and primary thyro-tracheal anastomosis is difficult and often biased by several parameters (grade of stenosis, glottic involvement, or severe comorbidities) that may influence the operation-specific and overall decannulations rates, without considering the outcomes in voice quality.

An overall decannulation rate of around 92% is reported in the literature after PCTR for severe grade III and IV pediatric SGS (**Table 2**). It should be noted, however, that early experience with a small number of patients usually yields better results because of the bias in selecting more favorable cases.

The Lausanne experience on 94 PCTRs for isolated grade III and IV SGSs and 47 E-PCTRs for combined severe glotto-subglottic or transglottic stenoses is shown in **Table 3**.

The most interesting feature of this series of patients was the analysis of time to decannulation, starting from the day of the first surgery performed in the authors' institution (**Fig. 14**). The predictors of less favorable outcome were as follows:

- Severe grade of stenosis
- Glottic involvement
- Comorbidities or congenital anomalies

Table 2
Published results of overall decannulation rates after pediatric partial cricotracheal resection for severe grade III and IV subglottic stenosis

Ranne et al,[17] 1991	7 of 7	~100%
Monnier et al,[18] 1993	14 of 15	~93%
Vollrath et al,[19] 1999	8 of 8	~100%
Triglia et al,[20] 2000	10 of 10	~100%
Garabedian et al,[21] 2005	16 of 17	~94%
Alvarez-Neri et al,[22] 2005	20 of 22	~91%
White et al,[23] 2005	87 of 93	~94%
George et al,[24] 2009	90 of 100	~90%
Total	238 of 257	~92.6%

Modified from Monnier P. Partial cricotracheal resection. In: Monnier P, editor. Pediatric airway surgery. Berlin: Springer Verlag; 2011. p. 315; with permission.

Table 3
Results of 141 pediatric partial cricotracheal resections (n = 94) and extended partial cricotracheal resection (n = 47) for grade III and IV laryngotracheal stenosis

Decannulation Rates	94 PCTRs		47 E-PCTRs	
	SGSa	SGSb	SGSc	SGSd
OSDR	42 of 46 (91%)	40 of 48 (83%)	17 of 22 (77%)	17 of 25 (68%)
ODR	46 of 46 (100%)	46 of 48 (95%)	20 of 22 (90%)	17 of 25 (68%)

Abbreviations: ODR, overall decannulation rate (after redo surgeries); OSDR, operation-specific decannulation rate; SGSa, isolated SGS; SGSb, SGSa + comorbidities; SGSc, glotto-SGS or transglottic stenosis; SGSd, SGSc + comorbidities.

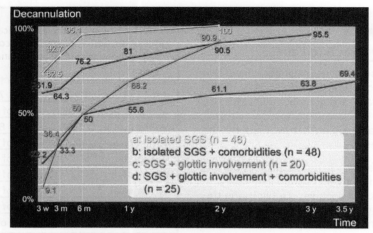

Fig. 14. Influence of comorbidities and glottic involvement on the surgical outcome of 141 grade III and IV pediatric LTSs. High overall success rates are obtained for isolated SGS (SGSa), albeit with a longer time to decannulation in the presence of comorbidities (SGSb). Decent decannulation rates are also obtained for SGS combined with glottic involvement (SGSc), albeit with more redo surgeries over a 2-year period. Poor decannulation rates, stagnating at around 68%, are seen when comorbidities and glottic involvement are present in the same patient (SGSd). In this last group of patients, failure to decannulate often results from comorbidities (swallowing problems, neurologic impairment, and so forth), although the subglottic airway is fully patent.

SUMMARY

Pediatric LTS encompasses a great variety of conditions that imply recourse to many different surgical managements. In that respect, preoperative assessments of patients and of the stenosis are key features to select the appropriate treatment of each individual patient.

Specific indications exist for

- Endoscopic treatments: fresh, incipient LTS and intrinsic, weblike, cicatricial SGS
- LTR: isolated PGS, minor grades of SGS and glotto-SGS
- PCTR: severe grade III and IV SGSs
- E-PCTR: severe glotto-SGS, transglottic stenosis, and congenital laryngeal atresia

In patients with and without comorbidities, overall decannulation rates of 95% and 100%, respectively, can be anticipated for isolated grade III and IV SGSs.

For severe glotto-SGS, these figures decrease to 68% and 90%, respectively. Severe comorbidities and glottic involvement (PGS, VF synechia, and transglottic stenosis) are predictors of late or failed decannulation, especially when both are combined.

REFERENCES

1. Bailey M. Congenital disorders of the larynx, trachea and bronchi. In: Graham JM, Scadding GK, Bull PD,

editors. Pediatric ENT. Heidelberg (Germany): Springer; 2008. p. 189–95.
2. Monnier Ph. Congenital anomalies of the larynx and trachea. In: Monnier PH, editor. Pediatric airway surgery. Heidelberg (Germany): Springer; 2011. p. 97–179.
3. Benjamin B, Holinger LD. Laryngeal complications of endotracheal intubation. Ann Otol Rhinol Laryngol 2008;117(suppl 200):2–20.
4. Cotton RT, Myer CM III, O'Connor DM, et al. Pediatric laryngotracheal reconstruction with cartilage grafts and endotracheal tube stenting: the single-stage approach. Laryngoscope 1995;105: 818–21.
5. Cotting J, Perez MH. Post-extubation respiratory care management. In: Monnier Ph, editor. Pediatric airway surgery. Heidelberg (Germany): Springer; 2011. p. 306–9.
6. Monnier Ph, Dikkers FG, Eckel H, et al. Preoperative assessment and classification of benign laryngotracheal stenosis: a consensus paper of the European Laryngological Society. Eur Arch Otorhinolaryngol 2015;272:2885–96.
7. Lambert V, Sigal-Cinqualbre A, Belli E, et al. Preoperative and postoperative evaluation of airways compression in pediatric patients with 3-dimensional multislice computed tomographic scanning: effect on surgical management. J Cardiovasc Surg 2005; 129:1111–8.
8. Monnier Ph. Endoscopic assessment of the compromised pediatric airway. In: Monnier PH, editor. Pediatric airway surgery. Heidelberg (Germany): Springer; 2011. p. 77–95.

9. Myer CM III, O'Connor DM, Cotton RT. Proposed grading system for subglottic stenosis based on endotracheal tube sizes. Ann Otol Rhinol Laryngol 1994;103:319–23.

10. Monnier Ph, Ikonomidis C, Jaquet Y, et al. Proposal of a new classification for optimising outcome assessment following partial cricotracheal resections in severe pediatric subglottic stenosis. Int J Pediatr Otorhinolaryngol 2009;73: 1217–21.

11. Monnier Ph. Preoperative assessment, indications for surgery and parental counselling. In: Monnier PH, editor. Pediatric airway surgery. Heidelberg (Germany): Springer; 2011. p. 231–40.

12. Bailey M, Hoeve H, Monnier Ph. Paediatric laryngotracheal stenosis: a consensus paper from three European centres. Eur Arch Otorhinolaryngol 2003; 260:118–23.

13. Alshammari J, Monnier Ph. Airway stenting with the LT-Mold for severe glotto-subglottic stenosis or intractable aspiration: experience in 65 cases. Eur Arch Otorhinolaryngol 2012;269:2531–8.

14. Pearson FG, Cooper JD, Nelems JM, et al. Primary tracheal anastomosis after resection of the cricoid cartilage with preservation of the recurrent laryngeal nerves. J Thorac Cardiovasc Surg 1975;70: 806–16.

15. Pearson FG, Brito-Filomeno L, Cooper JD. Experience with partial cricoid resection and thyrotracheal anastomosis. Ann Otol Rhinol Laryngol 1986;95: 582–5.

16. Sandu K, Monnier Ph. Cricotracheal resection. Otolaryngol Clin North Am 2008;41:981–98.

17. Ranne RD, Lindley S, Holder TM, et al. Relief of subglottic stenosis by anterior cricoid resection: an operation for the difficult case. J Pediatr Surg 1991;26:255–8.

18. Monnier Ph, Savary M, Chapuis G. Partial cricoid resection with primary tracheal anastomosis for subglottic stenosis in infants and children. Laryngoscope 1993;103:1273–83.

19. Vollrath M, Freihorst J, Von der Hardt H. Surgery of acquired laryngotracheal stenosis in infants and children. Experiences and results from 1988 to 1998. Part II: cricotracheal resection. HNO 1999; 47:611–22.

20. Triglia J, Nicolas R, Roman S, et al. Cricotracheal resection in children: indications, technique and results. Ann Otolaryngol Chir Cervicofac 2000;117: 155–60.

21. Garabedian EN, Nicollas R, Roger G, et al. Cricotracheal resection in children weighing less than 10 kg. Arch Otolaryngol Head Neck Surg 2005;131:505–8.

22. Alvarez-Neri H, Penchyna-Grub J, Porras-Hernandez JD, et al. Primary cricotracheal resection with thyrotracheal anastomosis for the treatment of severe subglottic stenosis in children and adolescents. Ann Otol Rhinol Laryngol 2005;114:2–6.

23. White DR, Cotton RT, Bean JA, et al. Pediatric cricotracheal resection: surgical outcomes and risk factor analysis. Arch Otolaryngol Head Neck Surg 2005; 131:896–9.

24. George M, Jaquet Y, Ikonomidis C, et al. Management of severe pediatric subglottic stenosis with glottic involvement. J Thorac Cardiovasc Surg 2009;139:411–7.

Laryngeal Split and Rib Cartilage Interpositional Grafting
Treatment Option for Glottic and Subglottic Stenosis in Adults

Wael Hasan, MB,BCh, LRCP & SI, BAO, NUI, MCh, MRCSI,
Patrick Gullane, CM, OONT, MD, FRCSC*

KEYWORDS

- Laryngotracheal stenosis • Cricotracheal resection • Vascularized composite autograft
- Rib cartilage interposition graft • Airway reconstruction

KEY POINTS

- A good understanding of the respiratory function if essential to determine the optimum reconstruction technique.
- Adequate airway reconstruction requires the creation of a functional airway that is able to maintain adequate ventilation with preservation of the mucociliary function.
- Tracheal resection is ideal for short segment stenosis where tension free end-to-end anastomosis is feasible.
- Airway reconstruction with a vascularized composite autograft is the minimal requirement for a complex functional reconstructed airway.

INTRODUCTION
Historical Perspective

The first tracheal resection on humans was performed by Kuester in 1884. The resection was limited to 4 tracheal rings or 2 cm, and extensive resection remained infrequent. It was considered to be an impractical procedure owing to expected tension risk on the anastomosis. Multiple synthetic materials were tried in extensive resections and were found unsuccessful; these include steel wire, silicone, and mesh.

However, Hermes Grillo was considered the father of tracheal surgery, revolutionized our anatomic understanding of the trachea, and described various techniques and surgical principles in his book "Surgery of the Trachea and Bronchi" in 2004. This better understanding of laryngotracheal pathophysiology and anatomy has resulted in more advanced surgical techniques and more extensive resections and reconstructive procedures.[1–7]

Etiology

The optimal management of tracheal stenosis depends on correctly identifying the causative factors in each case. Risk factors for the development of stenosis include high tracheostomy, cricothyroidotomy, prolonged intubation, and proximal

Disclosure: The authors have nothing to disclose.
Department of Otolaryngology, Head and Neck Surgery, University Health Network, University of Toronto, 200 Elizabeth Street, Room 8N-877, Toronto, Ontario M5G 2C4, Canadá
* Corresponding author.
E-mail address: Patrick.gullane@uhn.ca

migration of an endotracheal tube cuff. However, iatrogenic stenosis from intubation with an endotracheal or tracheostomy tube is the most commonly reported cause. In this type, the pressure exerted on the tracheal mucosa results in ischemic necrosis and subsequent loss of mucosal integrity. This can progress with bacterial infection of exposed cartilage resulting in chondritis or cartilage loss. Healing by secondary intention then begins, resulting in dense scar contracture and stenosis owing to fibroblast proliferation and collagen deposition.[8]

Relapsing polychondritis and Wegener's granulomatosis involvement in airway stenosis is long recognized. The incidence of subglottic involvement in Wegener's granulomatosis is around 20%. Up to 55% of patients with relapsing polychondritis have airway manifestations with high mortality rates of approximately 50%.[8,9]

ASSESSMENT AND EVALUATION
History

When evaluating a patient with cricotracheal stenosis, the most important clinical symptoms are the onset, duration, and progressive nature of the disease. The severity of the symptoms and their impact on the patient's daily living and quality of life are most indicative factors for active management and surgical intervention. A history of previous intubation and the coexistence of obstructive airway symptoms such as dyspnea, wheeze, or stridor should raise the suspicion of iatrogenic tracheal stenosis.

Physical Examination

Flexible fiberoptic laryngoscopy is the first and most available rapid in-office upper airway assessment. The mobility of the vocal cords, laryngeal sensation, and laryngeal inflammatory upper airway findings, with limitation, can be rapidly assessed and help to initiate the first steps in the management plan. Patients with findings on flexible laryngoscopy suggestive of an upper airway obstruction should undergo further evaluation of their entire laryngotracheobronchial tree.

Examination under anesthesia with direct laryngoscopy and bronchoscopy provides detailed upper airway assessment, allowing accurate disease and stenosis staging, cricoarytenoid joint mobility evaluation, and tissue diagnosis of suspicious findings, as well as anatomic abnormalities. During this examination, a clear documentation of the length of the stenotic segment is essential as well as the endotracheal tube size by which the patient is intubatable with minimal resistance while maintaining adequate pressure ventilation.

Pulmonary Function Testing

The peak expiratory flow rate is the most sensitive test for the diagnosis of tracheal obstruction and the peak inspiratory flow rate is the most sensitive test for detecting inspiratory flow limitations. In a fixed upper airway obstruction, both inspiratory and expiratory loops demonstrate a plateau effect. However, this plateau is only visible when the tracheal lumen is wider than 1 cm in diameter, making this test somewhat limited as a primary diagnostic method in the evaluation of tracheal stenosis.[10,11]

Imaging

At initial assessment, all patients with suspected airway compromise should undergo a plain radiography with anteroposterior and lateral views that include both upper and lower airway evaluation. Careful examination of plain films can identify signs such as inflammatory processes; signs of subglottic stenosis, tracheal deviation, or widening of the mediastinum that help to distinguish upper from lower airway obstructive pathologies.

High-resolution computed tomography scans with 1-mm fine cuts is the most commonly used imaging modality to assess the extent of the disease and to plan reconstruction. More recently, the advanced 3-dimensional reconstruction technology has helped to enhance anatomic understanding of the tracheobronchial tree and improved surgical and reconstructive outcomes in all the reconstructive domains.

MANAGEMENT OPTIONS

Presenting symptoms of patients with laryngotracheal stenosis vary widely. These symptoms can range from mild silent dyspnea on exertion to severe, life-threatening, acutely exacerbated events.

The management of this condition ranges accordingly from simple conservative observational regimen, to active endoscopic procedures, or, in more complex cases, open surgical resections.

The stage of stenosis determines the level of treatment required. The disease stages vary based on the degree on intraluminal narrowing, lesion size, and the involvement of other laryngotracheal subsites (**Box 1**).[12–14]

The goal of surgical repair is to create an adequate airway, achieve decannulation, and preserve normal laryngeal function—namely, speech, swallowing, and airway protection. For most early stage disease, and in the absence of acute distressing symptoms, the management of conditions that are refractory to conservative and

---

Box 1
Airway stenosis staging systems

1. Cotton-Myer

    Grade I: 0% to 50% of lumen obstructed

    Grade II: 51% to 70% of lumen obstructed

    Grade III: 71% to 99% of lumen obstructed

    Grade IV: 100% of lumen obstructed

2. McCaffrey

    Stage I: subglottic/tracheal lesions less than 1 cm in length

    Stage II: subglottic/tracheal lesions greater than 1 cm in length

    Stage III: subglottic/tracheal lesions not involving the glottis

    Stage IV: lesions involving the glottis

3. Lano

    Stage I: 1 subsite involved

    Stage II: 2 subsites involved

    Stage III: 3 subsites involved

---

medical therapy is classically attempted via endoscopic procedures. Failure of those is usually indicative of the need for more aggressive surgical resections, having no absolute contraindications present (**Box 2**).

Endoscopic Procedures

The endoscopic management of tracheal stenosis exposes the underlying healthy tissue where usually multiple radial incisions can be made in the stenotic area to facilitate its dilatation. This can be achieved using CO laser ablation,

---

Box 2
Contraindications to cricotracheal resection

Absolute

1. Stenosis at the glottic level

2. Active autoimmune or inflammatory disease

3. Stenosis that includes greater than 6.5 cm of trachea

Relative

1. Diabetes mellitus (microvascular disease)

2. Poor pulmonary reserve

3. Prior irradiation to larynx and/or trachea

4. Immunosuppressed patients (ie, high-dose steroids)

---

microlaryngeal instrumentation, or with scissors and biting forceps. The excision of scar tissue reduces the resistance to segmental dilatation of stenotic segments and it is currently recognized that the long-term outcomes of endoscopic pneumatic dilatation maybe superior to rigid tracheal dilatation.[15]

During endoscopic dilatation, the patient is placed supine in a snuff anatomic position. Ventilation is maintained using laryngeal jet insufflation or by tracheal stoma intubation. This technique also enables preoperative and postoperative airway assessment, with documentation of the maximum intubatable endotracheal tube size while maintaining pressure ventilation that enables obtaining tissue for histologic diagnosis, and the application of topical hemostatic, antiinflammatory, or fibroblast inhibitor agents.

The advantage of the pneumatic balloon dilators is that specific areas of interest can be targeted, minimizing the risk of collateral damage to surrounding tissue. The dilator is inserted when the cuff is deflated until the stenotic segment is reached. The position is checked before inflating the balloon, which is attached to an atmospheric pressure gauge that can be set to the desired intraluminal dilatation force to be applied.

Although this is a short, less invasive procedure with a minimal risk of postoperative complications, multiple repeated procedures are often needed over a long period of time. Outcomes, although variable, are less definitive than open surgical approaches, and limited to cases of early stage stenosis. However, this is usually not suitable for patients with synchronous laryngotracheal stenosis or with a segment length of narrowing of more than 1.5 cm.

Open Procedures

Tracheal resection

Tracheal resection is ideal for short segment stenosis, distal to the cricoid, where primary tension-free end-to-end anastomosis is possible. The cricoid level is the narrowest part of the adult's upper airway and, hence, the most common site for iatrogenic tracheal stenosis. Therefore, this procedure is more commonly indicated for the noniatrogenic causes, in particular neoplastic and inflammatory conditions. The preoperative assessment is critical in determining whether or not, after resection of the stenotic segment, there is sufficient normal trachea below the cricoid to perform the anastomosis. In situations where the stenosis is high, a laryngofissure may be necessary to facilitate the cricotracheal anastomosis.

Cricotracheal resection In one of the largest reported cricotracheal resection series of 80 patients, 92% were decannulated successfully.[16] Ideally, candidates for a single-stage cricotracheal resection are those who have not had a prior tracheostomy. Furthermore, an anastomosis closer to the undersurface of the true vocal cords of less than 1 cm increases the risk of cricoarytenoid fixation. The contraindications to this procedure are outlined in **Box 2**.

Airway reconstruction In 1991, McIlwain[17] demonstrated that the posterior glottis is lined primarily with respiratory epithelium that is in continuity with the subglottic and proximal tracheal epithelium. In the cadaveric position of the glottis, the posterior glottis constitutes 40% of the total glottic circumferential area and constitutes 60% of that area at full inspiration. This is achieved by 400% enlargement posteriorly with only 160% corresponding with the anterior glottic enlargement. The recognition of the anterior and posterior glottic respiratory epithelium lining confirms the existence of the physiologic and functional relationship between the 2 glottis sites and the respiratory system.

Tracheal allografts and aortic allografts have been used and reported. In a study of 14 tracheal graft cases using cadaveric processed tracheas, only 1 patient (7.1%) was successfully decannulated. In addition, this case series was associated with a high rate of postoperative infections (80%) requiring antibiotics.[18]

In contrast, although aortic allografts used demonstrated the development of respiratory epithelium after transplant, they were associated with a high rate of postoperative complication, infection, fistula formation, mortality, and lack of rigid support needed for respiration, requiring long-term intraluminal silicone stenting.[19]

A good understanding of the respiratory function of the glottis and subglottis is, therefore, essential when an optimum functional reconstruction of the glottic/subglottic area is considered. To maintain a functioning upper airway, a vascularized mucosal lining with a supporting rigid structure is required to maximize outcome.

At the University Health Network, University of Toronto, we have further enhanced our laryngotracheal airway reconstructive techniques over the years and now consider airway reconstruction in select cases with a vascularized composite autograft as the minimum requirement for a complex functional reconstructed airway. A retrospective study of 11 patients whose airway was reconstructed using a vascularized composite autograft between 2000 and 2011, after oncological and nononcologic resections, we reported no flap failure, successful decannulation in 91% of patients (n = 10), with the mean and median time from surgery to decannulation of 6.4 and 4.0 months, respectively. One patients had prolonged T tube insertion owing to recurrent granulation tissue, which required subsequent resection for a recurrent chondrosarcoma. All surviving patients had a serviceable laryngeal voice.[20]

Resection and Vascularized Composite Autograft Reconstruction: Single Institute Experience (University Health Network)

In a retrospective study, we report on 36 consecutive cases of combined laryngeal, subglottic, and upper tracheal stenosis treated with a single 1-stage procedure of circumferential resection of the subglottis and trachea with primary thyrotracheal anastomosis, combined with laryngofissure and laryngotracheal mucosal defect repair. This was a single institution experience; all oncologic cases were excluded from this study.

RESULTS

All 36 cases were performed between July 1889 and 2000. The mean age at presentation was 18 years (range, 16–72 years). Of those 77.7% (n = 28) were females and 22.2% males (n = 8; **Box 3**). There were 29 patients (80.5%) who were tracheostomy dependent at the time of referral and 27 (75%) had undergone previous surgical treatment.

Of the patients who had previous surgical treatment, 51.7% (n = 15) had previous dilatation with or without laser resection, 20.6% (n = 6) underwent prior open surgical procedure including laryngofissure, 3.4% (n = 1) underwent open scar resection, and 24.1% (n = 7) had partial cricoid resection and resurfacing of the exposed denuded mucosa using a buccal mucosal graft. In one of the cases, a total of 5 open procedures and 252 endoscopic dilatations were performed over a 10-year period at other institutions. Flexible and direct laryngoscopy assessment was performed in all 36 patients. Preoperative assessment included a high-resolution computed tomography scan.

The underlying etiology varied from postintubation injury in 80.5% (n = 29), idiopathic stenosis in 8.3% (n = 3), blunt trauma in 5.5% (n = 2), inhalation in 2.7% (n = 1), and congenital stenosis in 2.7% (n = 1). Of these patients, 94.4% (n = 34) had a significant reduction in cord movement limited to less than 2 to 3 mm and the cords were fixed in the remaining 5.6% of patients (n = 2).

All 36 patients underwent a single-stage procedure: 83.3% (n = 30) had isolated posterior

Box 3
Patient demographics

N = 36

Mean age 18 years

Male: female 3:1

Cause

Postintubation, 80.5% (n = 30)

Idiopathic stenosis, 8.3% (n = 3)

Blunt trauma, 5.5% (n = 2)

Inhalation injury, 2.7% (n = 1)

Congenital stenosis, 2.7% (n = 1)

Pathology

Isolated postglottic stenosis, 83.3% (n = 30)

Isolated anticommissure stenosis, 7.6% (n = 2)

Complete laryngeal stenosis, 11.1% (4)

Postoperative complications

Transient dysphagia, 58.3% (n = 21)

Temporary aspiration, 13.8% (n = 5)

Painful ulceration, 8.3% (n = 3)

T-tube migration, 5.5% (n = 2)

Successful decannulation

Isolated postglottic stenosis, 93.3% (n = 28)

Isolated anticommissure stenosis, 100% (n = 2)

Complete laryngeal stenosis, 50% (n = 2)

glottic stenosis and, of those, 86.6% of patients (n = 26) underwent a circumferential resection of the subglottis and trachea with primary thyrotracheal anastomosis, combined with laryngofissure and laryngotracheal mucosal defect repair with the pedicle mucosal flap as described by Pearson and Gullane.[16] In addition, 15.3% (n = 4) were managed by scar excision with lysis of adhesions and mobilization of the cricoarytenoid joints.

Of the 36 patients, 7.6% (n = 2) had isolated anterior commissure stenosis and were treated with simple scar division only, 11.1% (n = 4) had complete laryngeal stenosis, 3 of whom were treated with scar excision. The remaining patients had no identifiable glottic anatomy with both vocal cords entirely replaced by fibrous tissue that was managed by end-to-end anastomosis.

There were no postoperative major complications or mortalities. However, 58.3% of the patients (n = 21) had postoperative transient dysphagia, 13.8% (n = 5) suffered temporary aspiration, and 8.3% (n = 3) had painful ulceration at the lingual surface of the epiglottis owing to high

placed T-tube. Migration of the T-tube below the vocal cord was reported in 5.5% of patients (n = 2), which required replacement.

Of the 30 patients who had posterior glottic stenosis, the stents were removed successfully in 93.3% of patients (n = 28). The duration from removal of stents varied; with an average duration of 2 to 8 months in 86.6% of patients (n = 26), 14 months in 1 patient, and 38 months in the last one. Successful decannulation of 100% of patients (n = 2) with anterior glottic stenosis was performed at 2 and 5 months postoperatively.

In a group of 4 patients with complete glottic stenosis, decannulation of 50% (n = 2) was successful at 5 and 9 months; 25% of this group developed recurrent, severe cicatrical stenosis at the level of both glottis and subglottis, and remained tracheostomy dependent for a total of 4 years postoperatively, and 25% whose anatomy revealed no residual vocal cords were decannulated at 14 months.

HOW WE DO IT

In our series, a single stage procedure was performed in all cases, the steps are described herein.

Steps of Cricotracheal Resection

1. A standard collar incision incorporating the tracheotomy stoma is performed (**Figs. 1–3**).
2. The strap muscles and the thyroid isthmus are divided in the midline, exposing the airway from the hyoid bone to the manubrium (see **Fig. 1**).
3. The thyroid gland is dissected free from the trachea hugging the tracheal wall to avoid injury to the recurrent laryngeal nerves.
4. Identifying the recurrent laryngeal nerve is not attempted at any stage owing the usual significant scarring from prior surgical procedures to minimize the risk of iatrogenic injury.
5. The cervical trachea is then mobilized circumferentially beginning at the lower end of the stenosis and continuing upward above the inferior border of the cricoid ring (see **Fig. 2**).
6. The perichondrium along the inferior border of the ring is incised and freed completely from the anterior two-thirds of the cricoid arch (see **Fig. 3**).
7. Posteriorly, the perichondrium is elevated from the inner surface of the cricoid plate, which ensures preservation of the recurrent laryngeal nerve.
8. Dissection continues superiorly to the level of the inferior glottis and the diseased airway is opened in the midline via a vertical incision in the trachea and the cricoid cartilage.

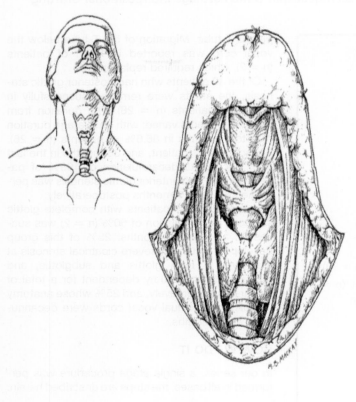

Fig. 1. The strap muscles and the thyroid isthmus are divided in the midline, exposing the airway from the hyoid bone to the manubrium. (*From* Pearson FG, Gullane P. Subglottic resection with primary tracheal anastomosis: including synchronous laryngotracheal reconstruction. Semin Thorac Cardiovasc Surg 1996;8(4):381–91; with permission.)

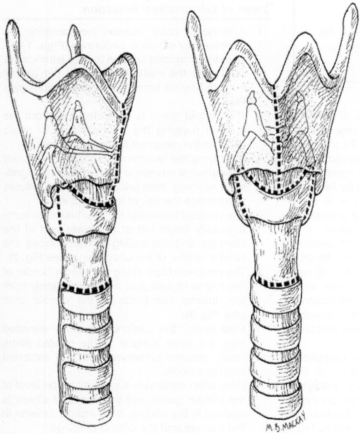

Fig. 2. The cervical trachea is mobilized circumferentially beginning at the lower end of the stenosis and continuing upward into the inferior border of the cricoid ring. (*From* Pearson FG, Gullane P. Subglottic resection with primary tracheal anastomosis: including synchronous laryngotracheal reconstruction. Semin Thorac Cardiovasc Surg 1996;8(4):381–91; with permission.)

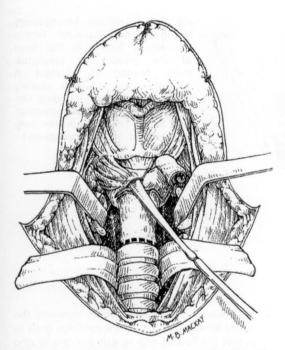

Fig. 3. The perichondrium along the inferior border of the ring is incised and freed completely from the anterior two-thirds of the cricoid arch. (*From* Pearson FG, Gullane P. Subglottic resection with primary tracheal anastomosis: including synchronous laryngotracheal reconstruction. Semin Thorac Cardiovasc Surg 1996;8(4):381–91; with permission.)

9. A laryngofissure is then performed to expose the glottic pathology.
10. Identification of the residual cords can be helped when viewing from below using the 70° rigid nasal endoscope.

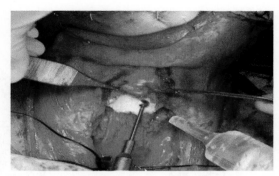

Fig. 4. Thinning of posterior cricoid plate using a #4 diamond burr.

11. The anterior two-thirds of the cricoid ring is then resected and the posterior diseased cricoid plate is removed with either a rongeur, curette, or burr, leaving a minimum of 50% of the vertical height of the posterior cricoid plate intact (**Fig. 4**).
12. The mucosa, submucosa and the perichondrium is then divided posteriorly above the level of the stenosis.
13. At this point, the degree of the laryngeal stenosis can be assessed and treated accordingly.

Steps of Defect Reconstruction Using a Vascularized Composite Autograft

After scar excision of the stenotic segment and exposure of the defect as described in steps 1 through 13, the following technique is used to reconstruct larger defects that are not amenable to end-to-end anastomosis (**Fig. 5**).

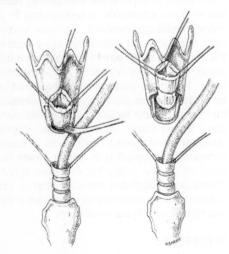
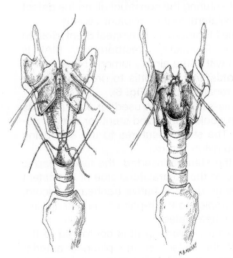

Fig. 5. Cricotracheal resection with a membranous posterior tracheal flap. (*From* Pearson FG, Gullane P. Subglottic resection with primary tracheal anastomosis: including synchronous laryngotracheal reconstruction. Semin Thorac Cardiovasc Surg 1996;8(4):381–91; with permission.)

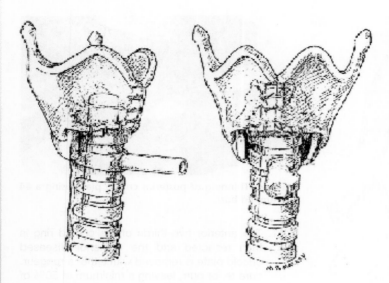

Fig. 6. A sterilized Montgomery laryngeal stent placed within the airway lumen at the level of the glottis and subglottis. (*From* Pearson FG, Gullane P. Subglottic resection with primary tracheal anastomosis: including synchronous laryngotracheal reconstruction. Semin Thorac Cardiovasc Surg 1996;8(4):381–91; with permission.)

1. A free buccal mucosal graft is transferred and sutured to the tip of the defect.
2. A temporoparietal fascial flap or radial forearm flap is harvested (the latter is preferred for larger defects).
3. Sufficient buccal mucosal flap and costal cartilage grafts are harvested to reconstruct and to resurface the defect.
4. The buccal mucosal flap is sutured superficially to the luminal aspect of the fascial flap with interrupted absorbable sutures. They will later become the intraluminal lining of the vascularized composite autograft.
5. The buccal mucosa and the fascial flap construct is then inset into the surgical defect by first suturing the construct along the defect side ipsilateral to the recipient vessels.
6. A sterile Montgomery Laryngeal Stent (Boston Medical Products, Westborough, MA) is placed within the airway lumen at the level of the glottis and subglottis to provide support to the reconstruction (**Fig. 6**).
7. A female-sized stent is used for male patients and an adolescent-sized stent for female patients. The stent is sutures to the skin using two 2-0 nylon sutures.
8. Once the stent is inserted, the fascial flap is sutured to the contralateral side of the defect and secured to the native trachea or cricoid, thus completing the repair of the anterior laryngotracheal defect.
9. The costal cartilage graft is contoured to the size of the defect or the planned anterior expansion of the airway and secured to the native laryngotracheal skeleton with interrupted sutures.
10. A sufficient gap is maintained between the native airway and the costal cartilage graft to permit the fascial flap to exit the airway and avoid strangulation.
11. The fascial flap is then wrapped around the costal cartilage graft and the vascular pedicle brought through a tunnel in the strap muscles.
12. The microvascular anastomosis is then performed, commonly to the superior thyroid artery.
13. The endotracheal tube is then switched to cuffed tracheal tube at the end of the procedure.

SUMMARY

From years of experience with airway reconstruction and the additional understanding of different pathophysiology involved, we now know that a rigid conduit lined with respiratory epithelium is the minimum requirement to maintain a functional upper airway and minimize long-term complications. The main goal of airway reconstruction is to resect the stenotic segment, maintain airway functionality, and facilitate successful decannulation. Single-stage laryngofissure, cricotracheal resection, and defect repair with a vascularized composite autograft is in select cases the treatment of choice today for complex synchronous glottic and subglottic stenosis that is refractory to conservative and minimally invasive endoscopic techniques within our institution.

REFERENCES

1. Ogura J, Biller H. Reconstruction of the larynx following blunt trauma. Ann Otol Rhinol Laryngol 1971;80:492–506.

2. Gerwat J, Bryce D. The management of subglottic stenosis by resection and direct anastomosis. Laryngoscope 1974;84:940–7.
3. Pearson FG, Cooper J, Nelms J, et al. Primary tracheal anastomosis after resection of the cartilage with preservation of the recurrent laryngeal nerve. Thorac Cardiovasc Surg 1975;70:806–16.
4. Pearson FG, Brito-Filomeno L, Cooper J. Experience with partial cricoid resection and thyrotrachea anastomosis. Ann Otol Rhinol Laryngol 1986;95:582–5.
5. Couraud L, Bichon P, Vally J. The surgical treatment of inflammatory and fibrous laryngotracheal stenosis. Eur J Cardiothorac Surg 1988;2:410–5.
6. Grillo H, Mathison D, Wain J. Laryngotracheal resection and reconstruction for subglottic stenosis. Ann Thorac Surg 1992;53:54–63.
7. Maddaus M, Toth J, Gullane P, et al. Subglottic tracheal resection and synchronous laryngeal reconstrucion. Thorac Cardiovasc Surg 1992;104:1443–50.
8. Foreman A, Johnson BT, Gullane PJ. Head & neck surgery book. Tracheal stenosis and tracheal neoplasms. JAYPEE - The Health Sciences Publisher. [Chapter 41]. 2015. p. 711–26.
9. McAdam LP, O'Hanlan MA, Bluestone R, et al. Relapsing polychondritis: prospective study of 23 patients and a review of the literature. Medicine (Baltimore) 1976;55(3):193–215.
10. Miller RD, Hyatt RE. Evaluation of obstructing lesions of the trachea and larynx by flow-volume loops. Am Rev Respir Dis 1973;108(3):475–81.
11. Miller RD, Hyatt RE. Obstructing lesions of the larynx and trachea: clinical and physiologic characteristics. Mayo Clin Proc 1969;44(3):145–61.
12. Myer CM, O'Connor DM, Cotton RT. Proposed grading system for subglottic stenosis based on endotracheal tube sizes. Ann Otol Rhinol Laryngol 1994;103(4 Pt 1):319–23.
13. McCaffery TV. Classification of laryngotracheal stenosis. Laryngoscope 1992;102(102):1335–40.
14. Lano CF, Duncavage JA, Reinisch L, et al. Laryngotracheal reconstruction in the adult: a ten year experience. Ann Otol Rhinol Laryngol 1998;107:92–7.
15. Lee KH, Rutter MJ. Role of balloon dilatation in the management of adult idiopathic subglottic stenosis. Ann Otol Rhinol Laryngol 2008;117(2):81–4.
16. Pearson FG, Gullane P. Subglottic resection with primary tracheal anastomosis: including synchronous laryngotracheal reconstructions. Semin Thorac Cardiovasc Surg 1996;8(4):381–91.
17. McIlwain J. The posterior glottis. J Otolaryngol 1991;(Suppl 2):1–24.
18. Propst EJ, Prager JD, Meinzen-Dierr J, et al. Pediatric tracheal reconstruction using cadaveric homograft. Arch Otolaryngol Head Neck Surg 2011;137:583–90.
19. Davidson MB, Mustafa K, Girdwood RW. Tracheal replacement with an aortic homograft. Ann Thorac Surg 2009;88:1006–8.
20. Rich JT, Goldstein D, Haerle SK, et al. Vascularized composite autograft for adult laryngotracheal stenosis and reconstruction. Head Neck 2016;38:253–9.

Distal Tracheal Resection and Reconstruction
State of the Art and Lessons Learned

Douglas Mathisen, MD

KEYWORDS

- Tracheal stenosis • Stridor • Tracheal resection • Suprahyoid laryngeal release
- Idiopathic subglottic stenosis

KEY POINTS

- Bronchoscopic assessment of condition of airway; that is, the extent of lesion and the amount of normal airway, is essential. Careful radiologic assessment is complementary and equally important.
- Careful collaboration with the anesthesiologist is essential to manage critical airways. Safe induction and emergence from anesthesia is essential to a good outcome. Patients should be managed to allow extubation at the conclusion of the procedure.
- Careful, precise technique is essential to good outcomes. Judgment is required to understand extent of resection. It is important to understand the principles to reducing anastomotic tension.
- Careful postoperative care is essential to good outcomes. Patients must be kept in mild flexion for 7 days. Flexible bronchoscopy is advisable at 7 days to examine for satisfactory healing.

It is indeed an honor and privilege to contribute to a volume on airway surgery dedicated to Griff Pearson. He was a true giant in this area contributing many creative solutions to difficult airway problems. He will be long remembered as a great friend and invaluable colleague!

—Doug Mathisen, July 2017.

INTRODUCTION

Tracheal resection is a relatively uncommon operation. The most common indication for distal surgical resection is tracheal stenosis resulting as a complication of prolonged intubation or as a consequence of tracheostomy. The injury from intubation results from an overinflated endotracheal cuff causing excessive pressure on the trachea and reducing blood supply. The resulting ischemic injury can be mucosal or the full-thickness of the airway, depending on the severity. Tracheostomy stomal injuries occur as a result of excessive damage of the trachea from technique, excessive traction on the tracheostomy tube, or infection. The pathophysiologies of these injuries are described in greater detail elsewhere. Tracheal tumors are uncommon. They can roughly be divided into 3 categories: squamous cell carcinomas, adenoid cystic tumors, and a group of benign or low-grade tumors. Whenever feasible, tracheal resection is the preferred treatment.

Symptoms

Patients with tracheal stenosis present with symptoms of shortness of breath of varying degrees. The degree of shortness of breath depends on the diameter of the stenosis. Slow growing tumors may have an insidious onset with shortness of breath only noticed with extremes of exertion. Over time, the stenosis progresses to symptoms

Disclosure: The author has nothing to disclose.
General Thoracic Surgery, Massachusetts General Hospital, Harvard Medical School, 55 Fruit Street, Founders 710, Boston, MA 02114, USA
E-mail address: dmathisen@partners.org

Thorac Surg Clin 28 (2018) 199–210
https://doi.org/10.1016/j.thorsurg.2018.01.010

at rest and frank stridor. Postintubation injuries usually present within days to weeks after extubation or decannulation. Recently extubated or decannulated patients who present with shortness of breath should raise suspicion of tracheal stenosis.

Initial Evaluation and Treatment

Surgeons initially treating patients with tracheal stenosis are responsible for diagnosis, initial management, and stabilizing the airway. In the nonemergent airway, computerized axial, sagittal, and coronal views of the trachea should establish the diagnosis in most patients. Initial management should include humidified oxygen and elevation of the head of the bed. Heliox and steroid administration can be effective in some patients who remain symptomatic. When a more urgent situation exists, it is best to secure the airway in the operating room. Control of the airway can be achieved by balloon dilation of strictures or dilation with bougies and rigid bronchoscopes. If a tumor exists, debridement may be required to establish a safe airway. Tracheostomy is a last resort. Care must be taken to place the tracheostomy in the proper position. Ideally, the tracheostomy should be placed through the damaged stenotic segment after dilation has been successfully achieved. This is to preserve maximum viable trachea for subsequent reconstruction. Ideally, a thoracic surgeon is best suited to control the airway with a combination of anesthesiologists, pulmonologists, and general surgeons. Once stabilized, the patient should have a thorough

evaluation. There is never a need for emergency tracheal resection. Patients who have been misdiagnosed with asthma and treated with high-dose steroids should be weaned and prepared for surgery after a sufficient period of time. After steroids are weaned, a wait of 3 to 4 weeks is preferable.

INDICATIONS

The indications for tracheal reconstructive operations are (1) primary tumors, principally adenoid cystic and squamous cell carcinoma, and a wide variety of malignant, low-grade malignant, and benign tumors; and (2) secondary tumors, primarily thyroid carcinoma, bronchogenic carcinoma, and, rarely, esophageal carcinoma. Benign conditions include (3) postintubation lesions, including cuff and stomal stenosis, tracheomalacia, tracheoesophageal fistula, and brachiocephalic arterial fistula. Other conditions include trauma, prior surgery, tuberculosis, amyloidosis, relapsing polychondritis, congenital malformation, mediastinal fibrosis, idiopathic stenosis, and Wegener granulomatosis.

PREOPERATIVE PLANNING
Radiology

The entire airway can be imaged with computed tomography (CT) and 3-dimensional reconstruction (**Fig. 1**A). Sagittal, coronal, and axial images are quite helpful in assessing the airway and are becoming standard. CT adds data about potential

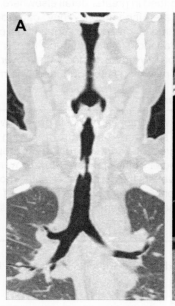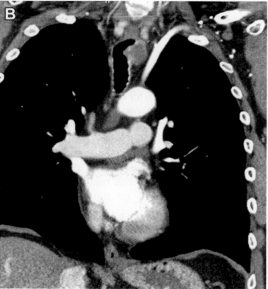

Fig. 1. (*A*) Tight midtracheal postintubation stenosis. (*B*) CT image with lateral tumor of proximal trachea.

mediastinal invasion by tumors (**Fig. 1**B). Knowing the location and extent of the uninvolved airway left for reconstruction is as important as defining the lesion itself.

Endoscopy

Bronchoscopy is essential but can be performed at resection unless the problem is unusually complicated. When laryngeal abnormality is suspected, the examination is often carried out concurrently with an otolaryngologist. Rigid bronchoscopy with general anesthesia provides better visualization of anatomy, superior biopsy specimens, and the potential for airway management and improvement through maneuvers such as dilatation or coring out of obstructive tumors. Measurements that can be used in planning an operative procedure can be made using the rigid bronchoscope. These measurements are the distance from the carina to the bottom of the lesion, the length of the lesion, and the distance from the top of the lesion to the vocal cords. The quality of mucosal inflammation can also be assessed. Care must be exercised in the outpatient setting when using flexible bronchoscopy to evaluate tracheal stenosis because of the possibility of precipitating airway obstruction.

Optimize Medical Condition

Patients must be in optimal preoperative condition to ensure a successful operation and recovery. Patients with postobstructive pneumonia, bronchitis, active mucosal inflammation, or those receiving high-dose steroids should undergo dilatation and the condition should be allowed to improve. Repeated dilatations may be necessary in some circumstances. Liberal use of saline nebulizers and antibiotics are useful to reduce secretions and inflammation.

ANESTHESIA AND AIRWAY MANAGEMENT

There must be close communication between surgeon and anesthesiologist. Each should know what the other has planned. Anesthesia for tracheal resection is best administered as total intravenous anesthesia (TIVA). This process provides satisfactory anesthesia and muscle relaxation before intubation, decouples ventilation and the delivery of anesthesia, and avoids environmental contamination of volatile anesthetics during the case. It also blunts airway reflexes and its effects wear off quickly at the completion of the operation, allowing for extubation. Remifentanil and propofol are delivered by infusion and are excellent agents commonly used with TIVA. The

goal is for smooth emergence from anesthesia and extubation at the conclusion of the procedure.

The surgeon should be available with an array of rigid bronchoscopes during induction of anesthesia to control the airway. A stricture less than 6 mm in diameter is dilated under direct vision with rigid pediatric bronchoscopes. For airway control at surgery, excessive dilation should be avoided to reduce injury and inflammation of the airway. If the stricture is greater than 6 mm, a small endotracheal tube (5.5 mm) may be placed through the lesion over a flexible bronchoscope. If the tracheal stenosis is located in the subglottic area, the lesion usually requires dilatation to allow passage of a small endotracheal tube. During resection of the trachea, the airway is divided, and the distal end of the trachea can be directly intubated with a sterile armored, flexible endotracheal tube (Tovell tube). Sterile connecting tubes are passed off the surgical field to the anesthesiologist. The Tovell tube can be intermittently removed for brief periods of apnea to allow careful and precise placement of sutures. This technique allows ventilation during reconstruction of the trachea. Before completion of the tracheal anastomosis, the oral endotracheal tube is retrieved from the proximal trachea and passed distal to the suture line. In many circumstances, it is necessary to secure a small red rubber catheter to the end and to the oral tube to allow control of the tube. Ideally, the patient should be extubated and breathe spontaneously at the conclusion of the operative procedure. This requires close coordination between surgeon and anesthesiologist. It is not desirable to have even a low-pressure cuff in close contact with the anastomosis for any period of time. If the patient does require intubation after surgery, a small, uncuffed endotracheal tube is preferred. The tube should be removed within 24 to 48 hours. If the airway is still a concern, a small tracheostomy should be placed 2 rings below the anastomosis. The innominate artery and the tracheal anastomosis should be separated from the tracheostomy by a strap muscle flap that is carefully sutured to the trachea.

SURGICAL TECHNIQUE
Basic Principles

Surgeons performing tracheal surgery should be familiar with the basic principles of airway surgery:

1. It is essential to preserve the delicate blood supply of the trachea. The blood supply enters the trachea in the midlateral position. Extensive circumferential dissection of the trachea should

not extend beyond the level of the resection. Preferably, no more than 1 cm of trachea should be circumferentially freed from lateral attachments beyond the line of resection.

2. Excessive anastomotic tension must be avoided. This requires experience, judgment, and an understanding of the limits of resection for different body habitus, prior treatments, radiation, tracheostomy, and previous operations. Skilled surgeons know whether they are attempting to pull the ends of the trachea together under excessive tension. Surgeons operating on the trachea must be familiar with all available techniques for mobilization of the trachea to lessen tension. They must also make a mature judgment in advance of resection as to whether sufficient trachea will be left to construct a safe anastomosis.

3. Precise anastomotic technique is required. Lines of resection should be cut cleanly. Fine absorbable suture material must be used. I use 4-0 polyglycolic acid polymer Vicryl (Ethicon, Inc, Piscataway, NJ, USA) suture for most anastomoses in adults, and 5-0 Vicryl in small children. Heavier 3-0 sutures are used anteriorly in some with calcified airways. Stay sutures are 2-0 Vicryl and are usually left in place after tying to reduce anastomotic tension. All sutures are oiled to promote sliding of the suture through tissues.

4. Surgeons should be familiar with all measures to reduce anastomotic tension. Careful sharp and blunt dissection of the pretracheal plane should be done. Traction sutures are used in all cases. If further reduction in tension is required, a suprahyoid release of Montgomery is preferred[1] (**Fig. 2**). Hilar and pericardial releases are sometimes helpful for very distal resections (**Fig. 3**).

5. The anastomosis should be airtight when tested under saline before coverage with a pedicled tissue flap. I cover all anastomoses. The strap muscles are ideal. It is essential to provide coverage if the innominate artery is adjacent to the anastomosis. Pedicled intercostal muscles or pericardial fat pad are used in the chest.

6. The airway reconstruction should function satisfactorily at the conclusion of the operation; extubation at the conclusion of the operation is the goal. If the anastomosis is not adequate at the conclusion of the operation, it is not likely to improve with time, with the exception of edema. If edema is suspected, a small, uncuffed endotracheal tube should be left in place for 48 hours. The patient should be given steroids for 24 hours, kept upright in bed, given Lasix, and their fluid should be restricted to reduce edema. After 48 hours, the patient is returned to the operating room and extubation is attempted. If the patient is still stridorous, a small tracheostomy tube is placed 2 rings below the anastomosis and a pedicled strap muscle flap is placed over the anastomosis to protect it, if not previously done. If concern regarding structural integrity of the airway exists, a tracheostomy is placed below the anastomosis. The anastomosis is covered and protected by a strap muscle. The tracheostomy is placed at least 2 rings below the anastomosis. Selection of the tube is critical. It should be long enough and big enough; it will differ in each patient. If patient is tracheostomy-dependent, it must be secured carefully to avoid dislodgement. In some cases, if uncertainty of the status of the airway exists, a mini-tracheostomy provides some security but is not a long-term solution.

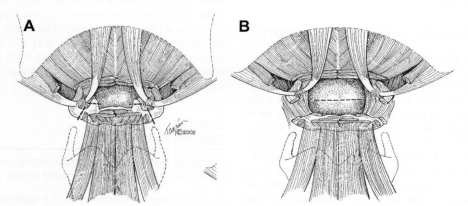

Fig. 2. (*A*) Insertion of muscles to hyoid bone. (*B*) The hyoid has been divided to complete the release of the larynx. (*From* Grillo HC. Tracheal resection: anterior approach and extended resection. In: Grillo HC, editor. Surgery of the trachea and bronchi. Hamilton (Canada): Decker; 2004. p. 543; with permission.)

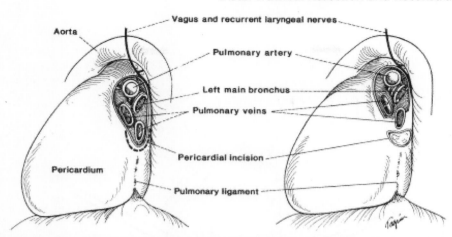

Fig. 3. The left-side intrapericardial hilar release technique, showing he U-shaped pericardial incision, which allows 1 to 2 cm of upward hilar mobility to facilitate the creation of a tension-free anastomosis. Dividing the pericardium completely around the hilar vessels gives additional release. (*From* Newton JR, Grillo HC, Mathisen DJ. Main bronchial sleeve resection with pulmonary conservation. Ann Thorac Surg 1991;52:1275; with permission.)

Anterior Approach

The anterior approach to the trachea is used for most benign strictures, even at the supracarinal level, and for tumors of the upper and middle trachea. The patient is positioned supine with an inflatable thyroid bag beneath the shoulders, to extend the neck. The head should rest comfortably in a soft device to keep the head from moving. The knee and hips are flexed to position the patient. A low collar incision is used for most operations (**Fig. 4**). The upper flap is elevated to a point above the cricoid cartilage if no laryngeal involvement is present (see **Fig. 4**). The lower flap is carried to the sternal notch. The anterior surface of the trachea is exposed. The dissection may be difficult and tedious in postintubation stricture with prior or existing tracheostomies, or when prior operative procedures have been performed. The strap muscles are elevated. The thyroid isthmus is dissected away from the trachea, divided, and retracted laterally with sutures (**Fig. 5**). An important element is to keep dissection absolutely close to the trachea so that the operator does not injure the recurrent laryngeal nerves while working laterally around the area of disease, where scar tissue and inflammation are maximal. No effort is made to expose the nerves because this would likely lead to their injury. Circumferential dissection is carried only a short distance above and below the lesion to preserve the lateral blood supply of the proximal and distal trachea. The anterior surface of the trachea is freed bluntly as far as the carina to provide mobility. If additional exposure of the distal airway is required, a partial sternotomy through the manubrium to the angle of Louis can be done. A

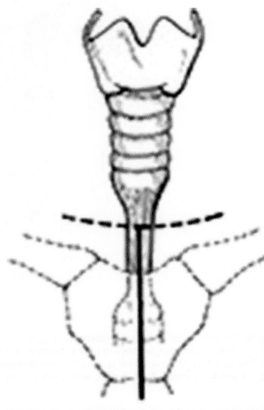

Fig. 4. A low collar incision is used for most operations (*dotted lines*). If more distal exposure is required for cosmetic reasons, a partial upper sternotomy to the angle of Louis gives exposure to the carina. A separate incision is preferable over the hyoid bone if a laryngeal release is required. (*From* Grillo HC. Tracheal resection: anterior approach and extended resection. In: Surgery of the trachea and bronchi. Hamilton (Canada): Decker; 2004. p. 525; with permission.)

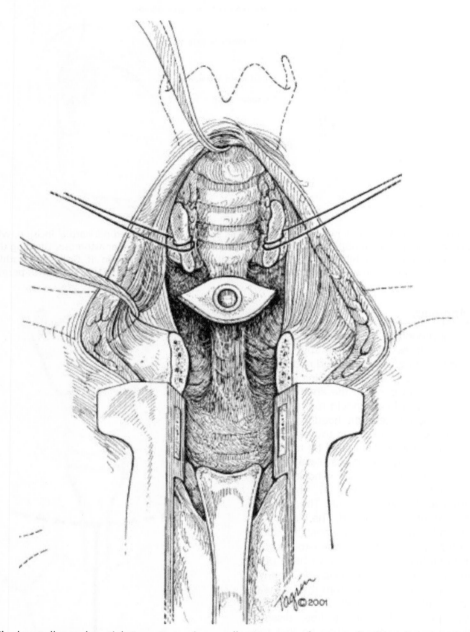

Fig. 5. The low collar and partial sternotomy give excellent exposure for more distal involvement. A small pediatric sternal retractor separates the upper sternum. Traction sutures pull the divided thyroid laterally. (*From* Grillo HC. Tracheal resection: anterior approach and extended resection. In: Surgery of the trachea and bronchi. Hamilton (Canada): Decker; 2004. p. 525; with permission.)

pediatric sternal spreader separates the sternum (see **Fig. 5**).

With tumors, the recurrent laryngeal nerves may need to be identified distal to the lesion and followed to the area around the tumor to provide a greater margin. If the nerve is involved, it must be sacrificed, although at least 1 recurrent nerve should be preserved. Adjacent tissue occasionally has to be resected with the specimen to provide adequate margins. This may include a lobe of the thyroid gland or part of the esophageal wall. Adjacent lymph nodes should be removed with the specimen; however, an extensive mediastinal node dissection cannot be performed without possible injury to the blood supply of the residual trachea.

With an upper tracheal lesion, it is important to identify the lesion. This can be obvious but if doubt exists the oral endotracheal tube should be pulled back, a flexible bronchoscope inserted, and the lesion identified by placing a needle through the suspected location and marked with a suture. I prefer to open the airway through the lesion so as not to sacrifice any usable trachea.

Traction sutures, 2-0 Vicryl, are placed at the midlateral position of the trachea on both sides through the full thickness of the tracheal wall and at least 1 cm below the projected level of division (**Fig. 6**A). With the trachea divided, the oral endotracheal tube is withdrawn above the lesion. The distal trachea is intubated across the operative field with a sterile flexible endotracheal tube and sterile connecting tubing, which is passed to anesthesia. An assistant holds this tube in position by arrangement of the lateral traction sutures, which can be drawn on to pull the distal trachea away

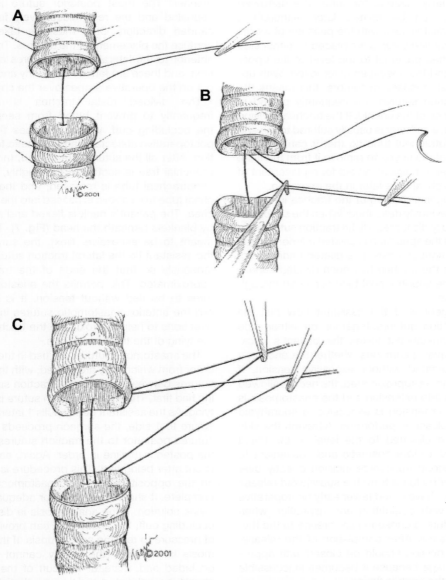

Fig. 6. (*A*) Lateral traction sutures have been placed. The first anastomotic suture is placed posteriorly in the membranous wall with knots ultimately being on the outside. (*B, C*) Each subsequent suture is placed inside the previous suture to avoid tangling when tied. (*From* Grillo HC. Tracheal resection: anterior approach and extended resection. In: Grillo HC, editor. Surgery of the trachea and bronchi. Hamilton (Canada): Decker; 2004. p. 534–5; with permission.)

from the field of dissection. The specimen is grasped with forceps and elevated, which makes the dissection of benign stenosis from the esophagus much easier. It also gives access to tumors that have posterior extension. If the esophageal wall is involved, either the muscular portion can be resected or the muscular and mucosal layers removed. For full-thickness involvement, the esophageal wall is then closed with 2 layers of interrupted sutures and covered with a strap muscle. This should be done over a bougie or at least a large nasogastric tube. The narrowed esophagus can be dilated later, although it frequently dilates itself with the passage of food.

Lateral traction sutures are placed on either side of the trachea proximal to the level of the upper resection and the specimen is removed. With upper tracheal stenoses or tumors, this means the lateral traction sutures are frequently placed in the substance of the cricoid. If the tracheal division is very high, a catheter is usually sutured to the end of the endotracheal tube so that it can be withdrawn out of the larynx to remove it from the field. The catheter remains as an aid for replacement of the endotracheal tube later in the operation.

In low lesions, division of the trachea is usually done as previously described. When the specimen has been fully dissected, distal traction sutures are placed and the specimen is divided inferiorly. If the lesion is a tight stenosis, it is dilated under direct vision after the trachea has been divided superiorly, and the endotracheal tube is placed through the stenosis.

The surgeon and the assistant now pull the lateral traction sutures together on either side while the anesthetist flexes the patient's neck. This maneuver determines whether the ends can be approximated without excessive tension. If the ends can be approximated, the neck is allowed to fall back into extension and the anastomosis is begun. If the tension is excessive, a suprahyoid laryngeal release is performed. Although the skin flap can be elevated to the level of the hyoid bone, I find it more cosmetic and convenient to make a second transverse incision directly over the hyoid bone to perform the suprahyoid release (see **Fig. 4**). I have noted fewer early postoperative difficulties with deglutition and aspiration when this procedure is chosen in preference to the thyrohyoid release. After completion of the release, the upper incision should be closed with appropriate drainage because it becomes inaccessible later when the neck is flexed.

Anastomosis is performed with interrupted 4-0 Vicryl sutures placed approximately 3 to 4 mm back from the cut edge of the trachea and approximately 3 to 4 mm distant from each other (see

Fig. 6A). The sutures are placed so the knots can be tied outside the lumen. I prefer to place all the sutures before completing the anastomosis. I begin with the most posterior suture in the membranous wall in the midline, placing each successive suture until the lateral traction suture is reached on that side (**Fig. 6**). This step is repeated on the opposite side to the level of the opposite lateral traction suture. The sutures are individually clipped with a hemostat, and further clipped to the drapes with a second hemostat in an orderly manner. The most posterior suture is clipped cephalad and the rest successively follow in a caudad direction. Care must be taken not to confuse the placement of the sutures. The sutures anterior to the lateral traction sutures are placed next, and these are fanned anteriorly and inferiorly out on the operative drapes over the chest.

The divided distal trachea is suctioned frequently to prevent blood from seeping past the occluding cuff, which increases the risk of postoperative atelectasis and the need for ventilation. After all the sutures are placed, the tracheobronchial tree is suctioned thoroughly, the distal endotracheal tube is removed, and the endotracheal tube from above is passed into the distal trachea. The patient's neck is flexed and supported by blankets beneath the head (**Fig. 7**). This is not meant to be excessive. Next, the surgeon and the assistant tie the lateral traction sutures simultaneously so that the ends of the trachea are approximated. This permits the anastomotic sutures to be tied without tension. It is helpful to pull the anterior anastomotic sutures in opposite directions to help approximate the trachea during the tying of the traction sutures.

The anastomotic sutures are tied in the opposite order from which they are placed, with the anterior sutures between the 2 lateral traction sutures being tied first. The excess of each suture is cut after tying. As the assistant gently pulls 1 lateral traction suture to 1 side, the surgeon proceeds to tie the sutures posterior to the traction sutures down to the posterior midline in order. Again, each suture is cut after being tied. This procedure is repeated on the opposite side. The anastomosis is now complete. It should be tested for adequacy under saline solution. If the anastomosis is distal to the occluding cuff, the anesthetist can provide 30 cm of pressure to test the anastomosis. If the anastomosis is proximal, the airway cannot easily be occluded and, instead, the cuff of the endotracheal tube is deflated and the anesthetist provides 30 cm of pressure while occluding the mouth and nose. Gas escapes through the larynx but, at that pressure, the anastomosis should demonstrate an air leak under saline solution if there is a problem.

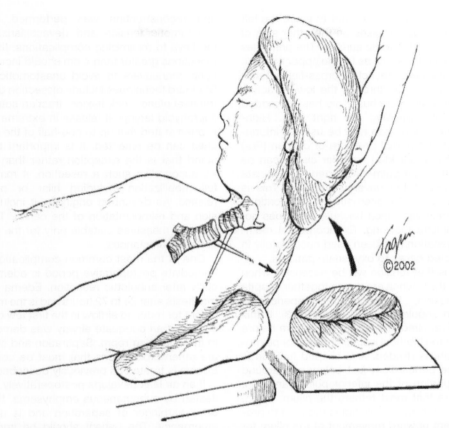

Fig. 7. Mild neck flexion is performed to assess approximation of the divided ends (*small arrows*). When all anastomotic sutures are placed, the neck is flexed and maintained in this position by 2 or 3 blankets under the head (*large arrow*) to aid in tying sutures with little tension. (*From* Grillo HC. Tracheal resection: anterior approach and extended resection. In: Surgery of the trachea and bronchi. Hamilton (Canada): Decker; 2004. p. 533; with permission.)

The anastomosis should be airtight. If a small leak is identified, it is repaired with 1 or 2 simple sutures. If a small hole is identified and cannot be repaired with a simple suture, a piece of strap muscle is carefully sutured and tied to the defect to provide airtight closure.

I leave the traction sutures in place, even though they penetrate the wall of the trachea. I have observed no difficulty with absorbable sutures. The thyroid isthmus can be reapproximated and the strap muscles sutured over the trachea. A second layer is preferable over the cervical and mediastinal tracheal anastomosis to protect the anastomosis and provide coverage if superficial infection develops. If the brachiocephalic artery lies directly over the anastomosis, viable tissue must be interposed. I avoid exposing the artery and attempt to dissect on the surface of the trachea rather than on the surface of the artery. In reoperations in which the artery is necessarily exposed, or in tumors in which the arterial surface

has been exposed, 1 of the strap muscles is sutured between the 2 structures. The wound is irrigated copiously and deadspace eliminated. A suction drain is placed. A chin stitch is placed to hold the neck in gentle flexion to avoid pulling on the anastomosis. This is not meant to be excessively tight or to sew the chin to the chest. Excessive flexion can create ischemia of the spinal cord.

Transthoracic Approach

The transthoracic approach is used for tumors of the lower trachea and carina. I prefer a posterolateral right thoracotomy, entering the chest through the fourth interspace. The azygos vein is divided, the pleura opened, and the trachea exposed. The vagus nerve is divided as it crosses obliquely over the trachea. If the dissection is carried high in the chest, care must be taken not to injure the right recurrent laryngeal nerve as it courses around the subclavian artery. In the dissection of the lower trachea, care must be taken not to injure the left recurrent nerve as it passes on the other side of the trachea over the aortic surface. The principles of resection are the same as for the upper trachea. If the distal trachea is resected, cross-field intubation is generally done through the lower trachea into the left main bronchus. This has the added advantage of collapsing the right lung. High-frequency ventilation can also be used. If intubation is used and partial pressure of oxygen (Po_2) begins to fall, a shielded vascular clamp can be placed on the right pulmonary artery to eliminate shunting through the unventilated lung. This is rarely necessary. An alternative is to continue high-frequency ventilation because this does not massively inflate the lung. Extracorporeal membrane oxygenation has been used successfully in highly selected cases to oxygenate patients.

If it seems that tension will be excessive when the ends of the trachea are drawn together despite cervical flexion, intrathoracic intrapericardial mobilization should be used (see **Fig. 3**). If this measure is required, it is easier to perform before resection of the tracheal lesion. The inferior pulmonary ligament is divided. A U-shaped incision is made in the pericardium just below and around the lower portion of the inferior pulmonary vein, the structure that most tethers the hilum. Often, this degree of release is all that is required to provide sufficient upward movement of the hilum for anastomosis. If this release is not adequate, complete circumferential division of the pericardium around the hilum of the right lung can be performed. When the pericardium is so divided, I attempt to save the pedicle of vessels and lymphatics in the posterior hilum by looping a tape around them. Salvage of these lymphatics may be important for the early postoperative function of that lung. The surgeon must remember that the neck should be flexed during the anastomosis because this delivers a considerable amount of cervical trachea into the mediastinum. Laryngeal release does not help free the trachea for distal tracheal or carinal reconstruction.

After the reconstruction is complete and tested under saline solution, second-layer coverage is provided with a broad-based pleural flap or pedicled pericardial fat carried in a circular manner around the anastomosis and sutured into place. A pedicled intercostal muscle can be used to cover the exposed aspect of the anastomosis. It should not be wrapped circumferentially.

COMPLICATIONS OF TRACHEAL SURGERY

Complications after tracheal surgery are similar regardless of the problem for which resection

and reconstruction was performed. Avoiding anastomotic tension and devascularization are the keys to minimizing complications. In general, resections greater than 4 cm should include additional maneuvers to avoid anastomotic tension. Standard techniques include dissection of the pretracheal plane, neck flexion, traction sutures, and suprahyoid laryngeal release in extreme cases. It is often stated that up to one-half of the adult trachea can be resected. It is important to understand that is the exception rather than the rule. To accomplish such a resection, it may require full mobilization including hilar or pericardial release. As described originally, it included division and reimplantation of the carina. These are extreme measures suitable only for the most unusual circumstances.

One of the most common complications in the immediate postoperative period is edema, especially after subglottic resection. Edema generally manifests after 24 to 72 hours and is the most likely culprit for reduced airflow in the first few days after surgery if an adequate airway was demonstrated in the operating room. Separation and secretions are other explanations that must be considered. Edema is treated as previously described.

If an air leak develops postoperatively, as manifested by subcutaneous emphysema, this could be a harbinger of separation and is a surgical emergency. The patient should be immediately returned to the operating room and the airway secured. In cases of separation, repair is unlikely and tracheostomy or a T-tube should be used to secure the airway. Local muscles can be used to buttress the tracheostomy or T-tube. If the airway is stable and the subcutaneous air is minimal, then CT imaging may be helpful in the initial assessment. Either way, the patient should undergo bronchoscopy to assess the competency of the airway. If a dehiscence is found, then surgical exploration and securing of the airway with a tracheostomy or T-tube is preferable. If the airway is secure and only a small leak from a suture or a small area of necrosis is identified, then attempted local repair buttressed by muscles using suction to press the flaps securely in the damaged area is often successful. Alternatively, hyperbaric oxygen therapy (HBOT) has been used to enhance angiogenesis, improve wound healing, and avoid reoperation.

The most in-depth analysis of complications after tracheal surgery was reported by Grillo and colleagues[2] in subjects with postintubation stenosis. The complications reported in this series of 503 subjects are summarized in **Table 1**. Granulation tissue formed at the site of tracheal anastomosis in 49 subjects in the series. After 1978, only 5 such cases occurred when the suture material

Table 1
Complications of operations for postintubation tracheal stenosis

	Major	Minor	Total
Granulations	11	38	44
Before 1978	10	34	44
After 1978	1	4	5
Dehiscence	28	1	29
Laryngeal dysfunction	11	14	25
Malacia	10	0	10
Hemorrhage	5	0	5
Edema (anastomosis)	3	1	4
Infection			
Wound	—	7	—
Pulmonary	5	14	19
Myocardial infarction	1	0	1
Tracheoesophageal fistula	1	0	1
Pneumothorax	0	3	3
Line infection	0	1	1
Atrial fibrillation	0	1	1
Deep venous thrombosis	0	1	1
Totals	82	82	164

From Grillo HC, Donahue DM, Mathisen DJ, et al. Postintubation tracheal stenosis: treatment and results. J Thorac Cardiovasc Surg 1995;109(3):490; with permission.

was switched from nonabsorbable suture to absorbable Vicryl. Thirty-eight subjects were treated with bronchoscopic removal of granulation tissue and 5 subjects required reoperation with a second tracheal resection. Four subjects required tracheostomy and 2 subjects were treated with T-tubes.

A total of 25 subjects had varying degrees of laryngeal dysfunction (aspiration or vocal cord dysfunction) after tracheal resection and reconstruction. Fourteen of these subjects had temporary laryngeal dysfunction that required no specific intervention. Eleven cases presented with more severe laryngeal dysfunction requiring either tracheostomy or T-tube. Two subjects in this series required gastrostomy tube feedings for persistent aspiration as a result of glottic dysfunction.

A total of 29 subjects had anastomotic dehiscence or restenosis. Seven subjects with this complication died. Two subjects had erosion into the innominate artery, resulting in death. Eight subjects with anastomotic dehiscence were treated with repeat tracheal resection with either good or satisfactory results. Four subjects were treated with permanent tracheostomy and another 5 subjects were treated with T-tubes, 3 of which

were temporary. Three subjects developed a dehiscence of a small portion of the anastomosis. Two subjects required reoperation and primary closure, and 1 subject was treated with cervical wound drainage and antibiotics. An additional 2 subjects required serial dilatations. Other complications included tracheal malacia, hemorrhage, and infectious complications, including 15 wound infections and 19 cases of pneumonia or bronchitis. In total, there were 12 perioperative deaths, 7 of which were related to the complication of anastomotic dehiscence.

Five hundred subjects undergoing tracheal resection were analyzed for anastomotic complications by Wright and colleagues.[3] Diabetes, resections greater than 4 cm, prior tracheostomy, age less than 17 years, and reoperation were identified as risk factors for anastomotic complications. When these conditions exist, special attention should be paid to reduce tension, optimize healing, preserve blood supply, and minimize risk of infection.

More recently, the use of HBOT has been studied as an intervention to enhance wound healing and avoid reoperation, tracheostomy, or T-tube placement in subjects with anastomotic complications after tracheal resection and reconstruction. HBOT is the administration of 100% oxygen at pressures greater than 1 atm and is thought to promote wound healing by increasing angiogenesis and collagen synthesis. In a recent series published by Stock and colleagues,[4] subjects with varying degrees of failed anastomotic healing, from cartilage necrosis to mild separation identified by bronchoscopy, were treated with HBOT. A total of 5 subjects underwent a mean of 13.2 HBOT sessions, which were administered in 90 minute intervals in a hyperbaric chamber pressurized to 2 atm with 100% oxygen 1 or 2 times daily. In addition, subjects were treated with broad-spectrum intravenous antibiotics, tobramycin nebulizers, and heliox, as clinically indicated. All subjects in this series had evidence of anastomotic healing within a mean of 9.6 days and none of the subjects required reoperation or tracheostomy after the initiation of HBOT. Complications were minor and included inner ear discomfort requiring tympanostomy tube placement, temporary blurry vision, and 1 subject who developed tracheal granulation tissue requiring bronchoscopic debridement. No subject developed a stricture requiring reoperation.

RESULTS

Tracheal resection and reconstruction for postintubation stenosis has proven to be quite successful.

In a series spanning from 1965 to 1995, a total of 503 subjects underwent 521 tracheal resections for postintubation stenosis, 13 of which were done for restenosis after the initial repair.[5] The amount of trachea resected ranged from 1.0 to 7.5 cm and was most commonly between 2 and 4 cm. Laryngeal release was performed in 9.7% of cases. Results were good (defined as an anatomically intact airway in a functionally normal subject) in 440 (87.5%) subjects and satisfactory (defined as subjects able to perform normal activities but with abnormalities such as stress with exercise, a paralyzed vocal cord, or bronchoscopic evidence of narrowing) in 31 (6%) subjects. There were 20 failures (4%) and 12 deaths (2.4%). Failures were treated with tracheostomy in 11 subjects, with T-tubes in 7 subjects, and with dilations in 2 subjects. Prior resection and reconstruction increased the failure rate from 3.6% to 5.6% and the mortality rate from 2.1% to 3.8%. The level of the airway anastomosis was also found to be a predictor of success. Trachea to trachea anastomoses were the most successful, with failure rates of only 2.2%. Trachea to cricoid anastomoses had a failure rate of 6% and trachea to thyroid cartilage anastomoses had a failure rate of 8.1%. Minor complications also become more prevalent with each level. Risk factors for anastomotic failure have been shown to include length greater than 4 cm, diabetes, age less than 17 years, preoperative tracheostomy, reoperation, and laryngeal anastomosis.

Careful patient selection and strict attention to technical details should result in very good results. First-time tracheal resection and reconstruction should achieve a good to excellent result in more than 90% of patients. Resection for tracheal tumors should have similar postoperative results.

REFERENCES

1. Montgomery WW. Suprahyoid release for tracheal anastomosis. Arch Otolaryngol 1974;99(4):255–60.
2. Grillo HC, Zannini P, Michelassi F. Complications of tracheal reconstruction: incidence, treatment and prevention. J Thorac Cardiovasc Surg 1986; 91:322–8.
3. Wright CD, Grillo HC, Wain JC, et al. Anastomotic complications after tracheal resection: prognostic factors and management. J Thorac Cardiovasc Surg 2004;128(5):731–9.
4. Stock C, Gukaysan N, Muniappan A, et al. Hyperbaric oxygen therapy for the treatment of anastomotic complications after tracheal resection and reconstruction. J Thorac Cardiovasc Surg 2014;147(3):1030–5.
5. Grillo HC, Donahue DM, Mathisen DJ, et al. Postintubation tracheal stenosis. Treatment and results. J Thorac Cardiovasc Surg 1995;109(3):486–92.

Factors Favoring and Impairing Healing of Tracheal Anastomosis

Farid M. Shamji, MBBS, FRCSC, FACS

KEYWORDS

- Tracheal and bronchial resection • Anastomotic healing • Surgical technique

KEY POINTS

- Circumferential tracheal resection and reconstruction requires attention to details of the surgical technique.
- Tracheal anastomosis after 3-cm length tracheal resection requires release maneuvers that will ensure tension-free anastomosis.
- Understanding the importance of preserving tracheal blood supply for satisfactory anastomotic healing is essential.
- Selection of fine needles and fine suture material for the anastomosis is essential.
- The importance of nutritional factors, drugs, metabolic disease, and irradiation affecting anastomotic healing requires vigilance.

INTRODUCTION

The understanding of wound healing from observation and scientific studies gained momentum when the importance of collagen synthesis and metabolism became recognized. This is reflected in further understanding of the gradual gain in tensile strength of the wound coinciding with progressive collagen deposition in the new granulation tissue forming in the wound during the first 4 days of the normal healing process. Decreased local tissue perfusion impairing wound healing was recognized early on when the pivotal role of unrestricted formation of new vascularized granulation tissue in the wound was recognized by pathologists. Microbiologists recognized the ability of infection to spread locally by lytic enzyme production (both by the bacteria and accumulating neutrophils) and that uncontrolled local infection could interfere with normal healing process by promoting collagen lysis over collagen synthesis.

Hence, the importance of establishing early effective local drainage of infection in the incision and near the anastomosis was emphasized. Historical recognition of vitamin C deficiency in tissue repair (eg, scurvy) was the impetus to study other nutritional deficiencies that could affect normal tissue healing. Over time, the role of vitamin A in wound healing and its beneficial effect in reversing the harmful effects of corticosteroids on impaired healing was studied. With increased understanding of radiobiology, the local harmful long-term effects of irradiation on different tissues and tissue ischemia became recognized and the concern was on healing of wounds.[1–7]

The publications in the *New England Journal of Medicine* in 1999 worth mentioning are on cutaneous wound healing and the interactive process of wound healing involving chemical mediators (cytokines) responsible for the phases of healing: inflammation; demolition of exudate and dead tissue; epithelialization, before formation of the

Disclosure: The author has nothing to disclose.
Division of Thoracic Surgery, The Ottawa Hospital–General Campus, 501 Smyth Road, Ottawa, Ontario K1H 8L6, Canada
E-mail address: fshamji@toh.ca

Thorac Surg Clin 28 (2018) 211–218
https://doi.org/10.1016/j.thorsurg.2018.02.002
1547-4127/18/© 2018 Published by Elsevier Inc.

essential new stroma, often called granulation tissue; and, finally, collagen deposition.[8–10]

To acquire a good understanding of healing of tracheal and bronchial anastomosis after resection it will help to look first at the necessary requirements. It begins with embryologic development of the tracheobronchial tree and histology of the wall of trachea and bronchi. Regional and applied anatomy of the tracheobronchial tree is the next step in learning. This paves the path for improved understanding of the normal healing processes in different layers of the walls of the proximal airways and the importance of protecting the blood supply. When well understood, it is possible to examine those factors that impair satisfactory healing of the anastomosis. Unfortunately, the standard textbooks of histology have not given in-depth histologic descriptions of the trachea, which would be of immense value to the surgeon.

REQUIREMENTS FAVORING SATISFACTORY HEALING OF THE TRACHEAL ANASTOMOSIS AFTER RESECTION

The most frequent indications for proximal airway resection are recalcitrant stenosis at the site of a previous tracheostomy and complications of prolonged endotracheal intubation; traumatic tracheal injury; selected tumors; and idiopathic strictures, particularly subglottic. Primary anastomosis is accepted as the preferred method of reconstruction following segmental tracheal and carinal resection. Mulliken JB and the late Hermes Grillo described the length of trachea that can be safely resected and reconstructed in the tension range of 1000 to 2000 g in detail. An average length of 6 cm of trachea (half tracheal length) may be resected and primary anastomosis may be accomplished safely by 3 carefully planned maneuvers: (1) careful mobilization of the trachea through a cervical or cervicomediastinal approach, (2) comfortable flexion of the patient's head between 15° and 35° equaling 4.5-cm tracheal length, and (3) intrapericardial mobilization of the right lung equaling 1.4-cm tracheal length.[11]

Satisfactory surgical outcome and healing of the anastomosis without complications requires careful patient selection, careful supervision of the trainees, and attention to the technical details. The requirements for safe tracheal anastomosis are outlined in **Box 1**.

Required Knowledge of Gross and Microscopic Anatomy of the Airway

It is knowledge of regional and applied anatomy of the larynx in the neck, and of the trachea in the neck and in the mediastinum, that are essential

---

> **Box 1**
> **Requirements for safe tracheal anastomosis**
>
> 1. Preservation of lateral tracheal vascular pedicles during tracheal mobilization
> 2. Tracheal mobilization should be anterior and posterior without inadvertent injury to the regional structures
> 3. Lateral tracheal mobilization should be limited to only the site of tracheal resection and within 1 cm of site of tracheal resection
> 4. Precise and sharp tracheal division and limited resection
> 5. Release maneuvers to minimize tension at the anastomosis before reconstruction
> 6. Careful handling of tissues
> 7. Proper placement of interrupted fine absorbable sutures 4-0 Vicryl sutures in the posterior membranous wall, followed by interrupted 4-0 Vicryl sutures on the anterior cartilaginous wall, encircling 1 tracheal ring on each side of the anastomosis that include the fibroconnective tissue between the tracheal rings on each side

---

in the conduct of a safe operation. The trachea is part of the lower respiratory tract, about 2 to 2.5 cm in diameter. It descends from the larynx at the level of sixth cervical vertebra, through the neck and thorax, to its bifurcation in the mediastinum at the level of the fourth thoracic vertebra. Its length varies with movement of the head and respiration but averages about 10 to 12 cm in an adult.

The walls of the trachea are formed of fibroelastic connective tissue reinforced by a series of 15 to 20 incomplete horseshoe-shaped patency-maintaining tracheal rings, about 2 rings per centimeter of trachea, united behind by fibroelastic connective tissue and smooth muscle where the trachea rests on the esophagus. The spaces between the neighboring rings are filled with a dense fibroelastic connective that is continuous with their perichondrium. This is a strong arrangement that enables trachea to remain a rigid tube and yet be pliable enough to be extended when the head is tilted back and enable the trachea to elongate during inspiration. The trachea is mobile, being pulled as much as 3 cm at the top and 1 cm at the bifurcation on swallowing. Its extrathoracic portion in the neck extends down to the sixth cartilage ring. The lower half of the trachea is intrathoracic.[12]

The tracheal wall is just 2 to 4 mm thick and contains 3 layers: mucosal, submucosal, and fibrocartilaginous. The mucosa is a pseudostratified ciliated columnar epithelium with goblet cells separated from the submucosa by relatively thin lamina propria set on a dense elastic lamina. The submucosa is a layer of loose areolar fibroconnective tissue containing numerous small mixed glands, with a rich blood and lymph capillary plexus. The fibrocartilaginous layer includes the smooth muscle in the posterior membranous portion, uniting the posterior ends of the tracheal rings. External to the trachea is loose fibroconnective areolar tissue (the adventitia) containing the nutrient small blood vessels and autonomic nerves that supply the trachea.[13,14]

Importance of Maintaining Safety in Surgical Technical Considerations

Precision in the surgical technique is of paramount importance to the successful outcome of tracheal surgery. It depends on the experience of the surgeon, who must pay a great deal of attention to the details of the technique and the principles of the operation required, appreciate the need to handle tissues gently, use fine instruments and sharp dissection, and ensure adequate hemostasis. Drying of tissues must be avoided and frequent gentle distal airway suctioning is essential. The selected absorbable sutures, 3-0 or 4-0 Vicryl (polyglactin 910) or PDS II (polydioxanone suture Ethicon), need to be placed at an appropriate distance from the margin: 3 mm apart and 3 mm deep on the posterior membranous wall and encircling first tracheal ring at both the proximal and distal ends on the cartilaginous wall. The selected suture material does not promote anastomotic healing; however, it should be strong enough to provide the necessary mechanical support for the anastomosis but fine enough to minimize trauma as it passes through the tissue. Likewise, the needle should be chosen so it will limit tissue damage at the tissue edge. As the anastomosis is completed, the adequacy of the lumen and viability of the tissue margins must be examined, and absence of tension ensured. The anastomosis must not be in close proximity to the innominate artery. If required, the adjoining viable thymic tissue or anterior pericardial flap can be interposed between the 2 structures. The use of omental wrapping with pedicled omental graft should be considered in the situation of compromised tracheal or bronchial anastomosis. It has the advantages of providing immediate sealant effect, controlling infection, promoting neovascularization and granulation tissue formation, and providing lymphatic drainage in the perianastomotic region.

Mandatory Preservation of Tracheal and Bronchial Blood Supply During the Operation

The first and foremost consideration is the preservation of tracheal blood supply during the operation so it does not to impair the flow of nutrients and oxygen to the trachea at the anastomosis. The blood supply of the trachea has been elegantly described by Dr Payne: in mobilizing the trachea before resection, it is essential to conserve as much circulation as possible.[15] At the carina, care should be taken to preserve the bronchial arteries. Although it is possible to clear and mobilize the entire anterior aspect of the trachea, care must be taken to preserve the posterolateral vascular attachments described by Dr Payne. In preparation of the divided tracheal ends for anastomosis, circumferential mobilization should be restricted to 1 cm or less (2 tracheal rings). It is well known that wounds with poor blood supply generally heal slowly with reduced tensile strength. Circumferential mobilization of the trachea must be performed with utmost care to preserve tracheal perfusion to within 1 cm of the site of tracheal resection.

The lateral vascularized areolar tissue pedicles of the trachea, which are very vulnerable to surgical mishap during mobilization, according to Grillo, must not be damaged during tracheal mobilization.[16] Any condition of persistent and chronic inflammation in the tracheal wall and immediate surrounding areolar tissue is liable to be accompanied by endarteritis obliterans and a poor blood supply to the proximal airway, as observed in the context of previous head and neck, and chest, irradiation (**Figs. 1–4**).

Emphasis on Tension-Free Anastomosis

Excessive tension at the anastomosis can impair nutrient perfusion and cause local ischemia of the tracheal wall at the anastomosis. Familiarity with all the tension-relieving maneuvers and specific applications in tracheal surgery is essential. In cases requiring resection of more than 3 or 4 cm of trachea, it is necessary to undertake mobilization procedures at the upper and lower ends of the trachea to obtain an anastomosis that is not under too much tension. At the distal end, the hilum of the lung can be freed by circumferential division of the pericardial attachments, including division of the septum between pericardium and atrium, which extends from the inferior vena cava to the diaphragm. This intrapericardial freeing permits resection of an additional 1 or 2 cm of trachea. A more extensive release is possible at the upper end of the airway. For this, the suprahyoid release described by Dr Montgomery[17] at

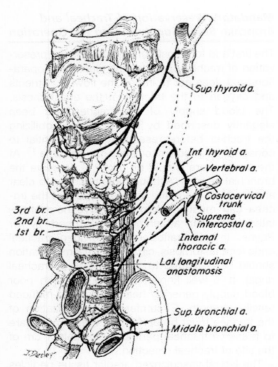

Fig. 1. Left anterior view of vessels supplying the trachea. The lateral longitudinal anastomosis links branches of the inferior thyroid, costocervical trunk, and bronchial arteries. a, artery; br, branch. (*From* Salassa JR, Pearson BW, Payne WS. Gross and microscopical blood supply of the trachea. Ann Thorac Surg 1977;24(2):101; with permission.)

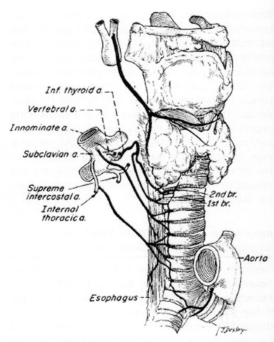

Fig. 2. Right anterior view of vessels supplying the trachea. The lateral longitudinal anastomosis links branches from the inferior thyroid, the subclavian, the internal thoracic, and the superior bronchial arteries. (*From* Salassa JR, Pearson BW, Payne WS. Gross and microscopical blood supply of the trachea. Ann Thorac Surg 1977;24(2):102; with permission.)

the Massachusetts General Hospital is frequently used. In this procedure, all of the muscles that attach to the superior border of the hyoid bone are divided, extending this division laterally to the level of the minor cornua. At the level of the minor cornua, the hyoid bone is divided vertically. Initially, the superior laryngeal release described by Dedo and Fishman[18] was used. This divides the soft tissue attachments anterolaterally between the hyoid bone above and the superior border of the thyroid cartilage below, down to the level of submucosa. Each of these release procedures permits resection of additional 2 to 4 cm of trachea. The suprahyoid release is a simpler technical procedure. It is not associated with the complication of transient dysphagia and aspiration, which are frequently seen with the superior laryngeal release procedure. During the postoperative period, unnecessary tension on the anastomosis is avoided by maintaining neck flexion for the first 7 to 10 days. This can be reliably and predictably achieved by application of a stout suture between the skin of the chin and the upper chest.

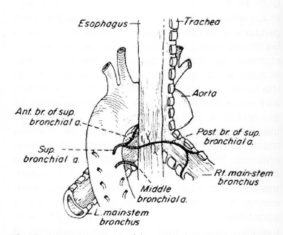

Fig. 3. Posterior view of bronchial vessels supplying the carina. The anterior branch of the superior bronchial artery and main trunk of the middle bronchial artery supply the lower thoracic trachea. a, artery. (*From* Salassa JR, Pearson BW, Payne WS. Gross and microscopical blood supply of the trachea. Ann Thorac Surg 1977;24(2):102; with permission.)

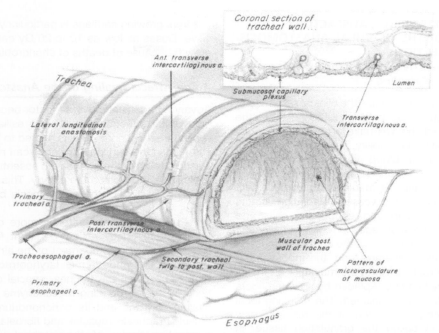

Fig. 4. Semischematic view of the tracheal microscopical blood supply. Transverse intercartilaginous arteries derived from the lateral longitudinal anastomosis penetrate the soft tissues between each cartilage to supply a rich vascular network beneath the endotracheal mucosa. (*From* Salassa JR, Pearson BW, Payne WS. Gross and microscopical blood supply of the trachea. Ann Thorac Surg 1977;24(2):104; with permission.)

The summary effect of all of these tension-relieving maneuvers permits an extensive resection, up to 7 or 8 cm of tracheal length, with a subsequently satisfactory primary anastomosis. The recommendations for the steps to take for tension-free anastomosis are outlined in **Table 1**.

Crucial Timing of the Operation

Tracheal margins at the level of the anastomosis should be healthy and, in this regard, the timing of resection and reconstruction may be critical in some cases. In the early stages of evolution of postintubation strictures, there may be extensive inflammatory changes in the tracheal wall and mucosa, extending both proximal and distal to the irreversibly damaged segment. Whenever possible, reconstruction should be delayed until these inflammatory changes have resolved. This may be achieved on occasion by removal of the indwelling tracheostomy tube and maintenance of the airway by intermittent bronchoscopic dilatation, or by stenting with a silicone Montgomery T-tube. It is equally important to be cautious when planning tracheal resection for idiopathic postinflammatory tracheal stricture until the inflammation has subsided; otherwise, the operation will fail and the stricture will recur.

Table 1 Maneuvers to gain tracheal length after resection	
Resection of Tracheal Length	**Maneuvers to Reduce Tension on the Tracheal Anastomosis**
Operations in the neck	
<3 cm	No special dissection and tracheal mobilization
3–4.5 cm	Neck flexion and chin fixation stitch
4.5–6.0 cm	Neck flexion, suprahyoid laryngeal release, and chin fixation stitch
Operations in the chest	
<3 cm	Divide inferior pulmonary ligament and mobilize the right hilum
3–4 cm	Previous, plus intrapericardial release of the right pulmonary artery and veins
4–6.0 cm	All of the previous, plus division and reimplantation of the left main-stem bronchus into the (right) bronchus intermedius

FACTORS IMPAIRING SATISFACTORY HEALING OF THE TRACHEAL ANASTOMOSIS AFTER RESECTION
The Adverse Effect of Radiation on Tissues and Impaired Healing

It is important to recognize the clinical response of normal tissues to ionizing radiation and the adverse effect this will have on healing capacity due to loss of tissue viability. The effect of radiation on micronutrient blood vessels is particularly important because late damage to many different tissues and organs is mediated to some extent by the effects on the vessels. Radiation affects proliferation of surviving endothelial cells and abnormal proliferation leads to regions of vascular constriction. Denudation of the endothelium leads to endarteritis obliterans and thrombosis, and capillary necrosis. In time, the muscular arterioles are gradually lost and replaced by collagen fibers and blood flow is diminished. The resulting local ischemia delays formation of the required new stroma, often called the granulation tissue, in wound healing that is a necessary step in all types of wound healing. The end result is atrophy, fibrosis, and delayed tissue repair. Unlike most hypoxic wounds, angiogenesis in irradiated tissue is not initiated from the existing vessels. Fibroblasts are most sensitive to radiation because many are in the G2 (second gap) through M (mitotic) phase and granulation tissue formation is impaired. Endarteritis obliterans from radiation damage cannot be reversed and cannot be restored by buttressing the anastomosis with vascularized pedicles. This pathologic damage has the consequence of impairing healing of tracheal anastomosis and there is no guarantee that buttressing the anastomosis with vascularized tissue pedicle can restore impaired tissue perfusion from the obstructed microcirculation. Under normal circumstances, regeneration of the arteries across the tracheal or bronchial anastomosis usually takes about 4 weeks. However, if nutrient tissue perfusion is previously impaired, the formation of the granulation tissue in the third stage of wound healing is delayed and likely to be inadequate, with consequent diminished tensile strength because collagen deposition is impaired.

Capillaries are very vulnerable and damaged by radiation doses above 40 Gy. Arterial damage occurs after doses of 50 to 70 Gy. The end result is ischemia of the irradiated tissues. This is an important consideration when tracheal resection and reconstruction is planned in a previously irradiated field because the tracheal anastomosis will be at risk of disruption. The effect of radiation on tracheal cartilage depends on the age of the patient. In children, growing cartilage is particularly radiosensitive. Doses as low as 10 to 20 Gy can slow the growth because of deaths of chondroblasts.[19]

Aging Affects Healing of the Anastomosis

Advanced age is an adverse factor because of its unfavorable effect on pliability and resilience of the hyaline tracheal rings. This is related to loss of tissue fluid in the cartilage proteoglycan matrix. The elastic stretch of the trachea, so essential in anastomosis, is thus lost in the elderly. This has implication in healing of the anastomosis because of excessive tension.

To understand this factor in more detail, it is important to briefly review pertinent features in the embryologic development of the airway.

Around the endodermal laryngotracheal tube destined to from the trachea, special condensations in the surrounding mesenchyme forms the hyaline cartilage and its perichondrium, smooth muscle (trachealis muscle), and fibroelastic dense connective tissue of the tracheal wall. Each tracheal ring is about 0.5 cm wide and 1 mm thick.

The hyaline cartilage of the tracheal rings develops in the embryo from the cells called chondroblasts that differentiate from the mesenchyme during condensation and begin to secrete the macromolecular constituents of the cartilage matrix. At the same time, the cells at the periphery of the site start to form a fibrous covering termed the perichondrium. The cells in the innermost layer of perichondrium generate new chondroblasts that deposit new cartilage matrix over the surface of that already formed. The cells in the outer layer of the perichondrium differentiate into fibroblasts that produce collagen and, as a result, the cartilage acquires an investment of irregular dense ordinary connective tissue that is known as the fibrous layer of the perichondrium. The fibrous part of the perichondrium persists into adult life. After chondroblasts have become deeply buried in the cartilage matrix, they are described as chondrocytes. The chondrocytes secrete intercellular matrix. The cartilage matrix is a resilient amorphous gel with a special kind of macromolecular organization. The gel consists mainly of hydrophilic proteoglycan, fine reinforcing collagen fibrils strong enough to withstand tensile forces despite being only 10 nm to 100 nm in diameter, made of type II collagen, hyaluronic acid, and water. Viability of the embedded chondrocytes ultimately depends on adequate diffusion of the nutrients through the essential tissue fluid component of the matrix. Moreover, cartilage is an avascular tissue, not provided with a capillary blood supply. The large volume of tissue fluid held in the interstices of its proteoglycan network enables nutrients and oxygen to reach its metabolically active chondrocytes by long-range diffusion from capillaries that lie outside the cartilage itself. Waste products are able to diffuse in the reverse direction to enter such vessels.[1] Nevertheless, total dependence on this very long diffusion path presents some problems, especially if insoluble calcium salts have been deposited in the matrix or from damage by ionizing radiation. This will have implications in the healing of tracheal anastomosis. Aging affects the pliability and resilience of the cartilage through loss of tissue fluid in the gel-like cartilage proteoglycan matrix and, consequently, in the healing of the tracheal anastomosis.

Local Sepsis Interferes with Anastomotic Healing and Tensile Strength

Local infection interferes with wound and anastomotic healing by release of collagen lytic enzymes and by creating an imbalance between collagen lysis and collagen synthesis. This interferes with the expected gain in tensile strength of the anastomosis.

Miscellaneous Harmful Factors That Impair Anastomotic Healing

An early and significant postoperative decrease in the suture-holding ability of anastomotic tissue occurs in the trachea and bronchi. This is reflected in the decreased breaking strength of the anastomosis. This loss in tensile strength is a reflection of an imbalance between collagen synthesis and collagen lysis, and usually occurs in the first 3 days of healing. The collagen lysis is known to exceed collagen synthesis in the presence of contamination and local sepsis, promoting increased accumulation of granulocytes and their collagenolytic activity.

The trachea is invested with a layer of loose areolar connective tissue, providing intimate support for tracheal perfusion, nourishment, and innervation. It is also the usual location for the process of inflammation, which commonly occurs during bacterial infection or autoimmune process, or complicating histoplasmosis. The ensuing mediastinal fibrosis, besides increasing vulnerability to damage to tracheal microcirculation during tracheal mobilization for resection and reconstruction, will prevent adequate tracheal mobilization for tension-free anastomosis.

It is questionable whether aging produces intrinsic physiologic changes that result in delayed or impaired tracheal anastomotic healing. It is more important to consider, besides older age, the presence of underlying disease that contributes to impaired healing in the elderly, including cardiovascular disease; metabolic diseases, such as malnutrition, vitamin A and C deficiencies, and diabetes mellitus; and cancer; as well as medications. Vitamin C (ascorbic acid) is essential to the process of anastomotic healing because it has a role in procollagen secretion from the smooth muscle into the extracellular space. Abnormalities associated with uncontrolled diabetes mellitus, which adversely affect healing, include prolonged inflammation, impaired neovascularization, decreased collagen synthesis, increased levels of proteinases, and defective macrophage function.

Low oxygen tension has a profoundly deleterious effect on tracheal anastomotic healing. Fibroplasia is significantly impaired by local hypoxia. Optimal collagen synthesis requires oxygen as a cofactor for the hydroxylation steps. Major factors affecting local oxygen delivery include hypoperfusion, local vasoconstriction, and excessive tension on tissue.

Large doses or chronic use of corticosteroids reduce collagen synthesis and wound strength. The major effect of steroids is to inhibit the first inflammatory phase of wound healing, including angiogenesis, neutrophil and macrophage migration, fibroblast proliferation, and release of lysosomal enzymes. Steroids used after the first 3 to 4 days postinjury do not affect wound healing as severely as when they are used in the immediate postoperative period. In addition to their effect on collagen synthesis, steroids also inhibit epithelialization, wound contraction, and contribute to increased rates of wound infection. Supplemental vitamin A helps reverse impairment of healing induced by corticosteroids. Uncontrolled diabetes mellitus contributes to increased rates of wound infection, reduced inflammation, angiogenesis, and collagen synthesis.[20]

The trachea may be affected in its course in the mediastinum by idiopathic fibromatosis that are known to manifest with Riedel thyroiditis, mediastinal fibrosis, fibrothorax, diffuse tracheal mucosal inflammatory granulations, retroperitoneal fibrosis, and obstructive renal failure. Mediastinal fibrosis may occur for other reasons, such as histoplasmosis, radiation therapy, autoimmune disorders, suppurative mediastinitis, esophagectomy, and mediastinal operation. These make safe mobilization for tracheal resection and tension-free reconstruction not possible.

SUMMARY

Integrated knowledge of the regional and applied anatomy of the human trachea in the neck and

Table 2
Factors influencing healing of tracheal anastomosis

Local: Favorable Surgical Factors	Systemic: Adverse Factors
1. Avoid interference with tracheal blood supply during tracheal mobilization 2. Minimize tension on tracheal anastomosis 3. Preserve viable healthy tissue edges at the anastomosis 4. Protect against local bacterial contamination and sepsis 5. Viable tissue pedicle wrapping supports anastomotic healing 6. Select fine absorbable suture on fine atraumatic needle for anastomosis 7. Use proper suturing technique	Patient factors 1. Advanced age 2. Chronic steroid therapy 3. Diabetes mellitus 4. Autoimmune disease 5. Malnutrition: protein, vitamins A and C, and trace element zinc 6. Cigarette tobacco smoking 7. Cancer 8. Medications Disease factors 1. Preoperative radiation to the neck and chest 2. Chronic active tracheal mucosal inflammatory process 3. Idiopathic and acquired mediastinal fibrosis 4. Previous tracheal resection 5. Previous mediastinal operation of esophagus, ascending aorta, or tumor 6. Incorrect diagnosis

From Waldhausen JA, Pierce WS. Johnson's surgery of the chest. St Louis: Mosby; 1996. p. 186; with permission.

the mediastinum, histology and the physiology of the trachea, diseases that affect the trachea, normal wound healing process, and favorable and adverse factors on healing of the tracheal anastomosis are required for the successful outcome of tracheal resection and reconstruction, as well as carinal resection and reconstruction (**Table 2**).

REFERENCES

1. Newcombe JF. Wound healing [Chapter 26]. In: Irvine WT, editor. Scientific Basis of Surgery. Churchill Livingstone; 1972. p. 433–56.
2. Singer AJ, Clark RAF. Cutaneous wound healing. N Engl J Med 1999;341(10):738–46.
3. Witte MA, Barbul A. General principles of wound healing. Surg Clin North Am 1997;77(3):509–28.
4. Thornton FJ, Barbul A. Healing in the gastrointestinal tract. Surg Clin North Am 1997;77(3):549–73.
5. Hunt TK. Disorders of wound healing. World J Surg 1980;4:271–7.
6. Williams JZ, Barbul A. Nutrition and wound healing. Surg Clin North Am 2003;83:571–96.
7. Townsend CM, Beauchamp RD, Evers RM, et al. Sabiston textbook of surgery [Chapter 8]. Saunders Elsevier; 2008. p. 191–216.
8. Grant ME, Prockop DJ. The biosynthesis of collagen. 1. N Engl J Med 1972;286(4):194–9.
9. Grant ME, Prockop DJ. The biosynthesis of collagen. 2. N Engl J Med 1972;286(5):242–9.
10. Grant ME, Prockop DJ. The biosynthesis of collagen. 3. N Engl J Med 1972;286(6):291–300.
11. Mulliken JB, Grillo HC. The limits of tracheal resection with primary anastomosis. J Thorac Cardiovasc Surg 1968;55(3):418–21.
12. Romanes G J. Cunningham's textbook of anatomy. In: Wyburn GM, editor. The respiratory system. 10th edition. London University Press; 1964. p. 447–73.
13. Cormack DH. Ham's histology, 9th edition [Chapter 11]. Lippincott; 1987.
14. Leeson CR, Leeson TS, Paparo AA. Textbook of histology, 5th Edition. WB Saunders Company; 1985. p. 382–408.
15. Salassa JR, Pearson BW, Spencer Payne W. Gross and microscopical blood supply of the trachea. Ann Thorac Surg 1977;24(2):100–7.
16. Miura T, Grillo HC. The contribution of the inferior thyroid artery to the blood supply of the human trachea. Surg Gynecol Obstet 1966;123:99–102.
17. Montgomery WW. Suprahyoid release for tracheal anastomosis. Arch Otolaryngol 1974;99:255–60.
18. Dedo HH, Fishman NH. Laryngeal release and sleeve resection for tracheal stenosis. Ann Otol Rhinol Laryngol 1969;78:285–96.
19. Hall EJ, Giaccia A J. Radiobiology for the radiologist, 7th edition. Lippincott and Williams&Wilkins; 2010. p. 327–55.
20. Ehrlich HP, Hunt TK. Effects of cortisone and vitamin A on wound healing. Ann Surg 1968;167(3):324–8.

Airway Management Following Tracheal Surgery

Thomas R.J. Todd, MD, FRCSC*

KEYWORDS

- Trachea • Ventilation • Bronchoscopy • Respiratory failure • "T" tube

KEY POINTS

- Prophylactic measures and careful monitoring of the patient in the early postoperative period may help prevent the onset of respiratory failure following resections of the airway.
- Bronchoscopic monitoring of the airway to assess anastomotic healing, secretion retention, and "T"-tube position is extremely important.
- The intubation of the patient following tracheal surgery is best achieved with the assistance of a bronchoscope, and the technique used will depend on the presence or absence of a "T" tube and the level of the anastomosis.
- There are a variety of techniques for ventilating the patient depending on pulmonary compliance, the presence of a "T" tube, and the ability to secure a leak-free system.

INTRODUCTION

Griff Pearson was a master surgeon, and it was the author's privilege not only to be one of his trainees but also to practice as his partner for 22 years. During that time it became clear that, although he was passionate about all forms of Thoracic Surgery, surgery of the trachea held a special place in his heart. As a Thoracic Surgeon but also critical care specialist, the author found this cadre of patients was especially interesting and presented opportunities to learn much about the management of the difficult airway.

What follows is the result of the experience gained during that time period and as a result represents the author's personal experience. Indeed, there is very little literature available on the subject of airway management once either airway compromise or respiratory failure ensues following tracheal resection. The author's and Dr Pearson's relatively large experience in tracheal surgery at Toronto General Hospital (now University Health Network) allowed them to experience most of the airway complications that can ensue following this highly specialized surgery. As such, they learned from trial and error what seemed to be the most successful solution to difficulties as they arose. As Hermes Grillo and colleagues[1] noted in their 1986 summary of a lifetime of experience, the results their patients experienced in the latter half of this large tracheal practice were superior to that noted in the first cohorts of patients.[1]

IN THE OPERATING ROOM

The postoperative management of the airway begins in the operating room. Tracheal surgeons agree that it is optimal if extubation is performed in the operating room at the end of the procedure. A high success rate for early extubation depends on several factors, not the least of which is close communication between the surgeon and anesthetist. In particular, once the airway is closed with a completed anastomosis, the anesthetist

Disclosure: The author has nothing to disclose.
The Canadian Medical Protective Association, PO Box 8225, Station T, Ottawa, ON K1G3H7, Canada
* 9 Lewis Street, Perth, Ontario K7H1M6, Canada.
E-mail address: ttodd@cmpa.org

needs to begin reversal of anesthesia to ensure that the patient is breathing spontaneously once the procedure has concluded. At the same time, however, sedation must be sufficient to avoid the patient excessively struggling against the tube. Prevention of excessive struggling will be particularly important during routine bronchoscopy, as is noted in later discussion.

The procedure ends with the application of the "chin stitch," a heavy suture applied in the submental groove and the manubrial-sternal junction in order to keep the neck in exaggerated flexion, hence decreasing anastomotic tension. The author's practice was always to have the anesthetist provide 10 to 15 mL of 2% lidocaine down the endotracheal tube as the chin stitch was being completed. This dose of lidocaine provides sufficient local anesthetic to the airway to permit the routine flexible bronchoscopic evaluation of the airway, which is undertaken before attempted extubation without the patient coughing or bucking during the procedure.

Flexible bronchoscopy through the endotracheal tube is an important adjunct to postoperative airway management. It permits the surgeon to evaluate the anastomosis for patency. In addition, it facilitates a thorough clearing of airway secretions, which along with blood will likely have accumulated throughout the resection. In addition, it is not infrequent, especially with cricoid and long segmental resections for a silicone T tube to have been inserted at the conclusion of the anastomosis.[2] Bronchoscopic assessment to ensure the tube is not kinked or twisted is essential. Bronchoscopy also provides the best assessment of the T-tube (Boston Medical Products, Westborough, MA) position relative to the vocal cords, the anastomosis, and the tracheal carina. Many surgeons will undertake such a bronchoscopic assessment of the T tube immediately following its insertion and before closure of the incision. On occasion, the tube will require readjustment based on this evaluation. It was the author's practice to assess the T-tube position after its insertion and undertake a thorough cleaning of the distal airway at that time. In addition, the author found it important to repeat the procedure once the chin stitch had been applied and as the endotracheal tube was being removed. This second bronchoscopy permitted a further assessment of pooled secretions and blood in the airway but also the opportunity to ensure that the T tube was not kinked from cervical flexion as well as to assess the vocal cords as the endotracheal tube exited the airway. The latter assessment is particularly important following subglottic resections involving removal of the posterior cricoid plate because considerable glottic edema may already be present.

There may be occasions when extubation in the operating room is not feasible. Such may be secondary to an inadequate reversal of anesthesia and thus poor respiratory effort. Glottic edema and retained secretions may also not permit extubation. Under such circumstances, the author would agree with Auchincloss and Wright[3] that it is best to place a small (6.5–7.0 mm) uncuffed endotracheal tube beyond the anastomosis. Such is best inserted under flexible bronchoscopic guidance to avoid trauma to the fresh tracheal suture line (see later discussion for technical considerations). The author prefers a nasotracheal tube under such circumstances when the neck is in hyperflexion because the ability to adequately view the glottis and angle the endotracheal tube through the cords is enhanced. Following laryngotracheal resection, D'Andrilli and colleagues[4] routinely leave such a nasotracheal tube in place for 24 hours; this permits them to extubate after another airway suctioning with the patient fully awake and breathing spontaneously, although such has not been the practice in Toronto. Should a nasotracheal tube be left in place for 24 hours or more, it is best for the patient to be returned to the operating room for endotracheal tube removal with anesthesia present so that all options are available should any difficulty with the airway be encountered.

IN THE INTENSIVE CARE UNIT/STEP-DOWN UNIT
Observation and Monitoring

As the heading suggests, the first few days following tracheal reconstruction are best managed in a specialized unit where expertise in airway management can be provided. Familiarity of the staff, especially nursing and physiotherapy, is essential in order to prevent airway compromise in those first postoperative days. Glottic and subglottic edema can be problematic, especially if the subglottic area has been transgressed or if a laryngeal release was required to reduce anastomotic tension. One can usually anticipate that the swelling will plateau at 72 hours. Airway secretions will be excessive for several days, and the patient's ability to adequately clear the airway will be compromised. Not only will secretions be increased, but there is also a reasonable chance that there will be retained blood and fluid in the distal airway despite the efforts of bronchoscopy in the immediate postoperative period. Glottic edema, postoperative pain, and the hyper neck flexion required in the more major resections to avoid anastomotic tension all conspire to reduce the patient's ability to cough and clear the airway of secretions.

As a result, close monitoring of respiratory function is very important, so that intervention to reestablish a patent airway can be undertaken before an emergency ensues. Constant oxygen saturation monitoring and frequent arterial blood gas assessment are extremely important. Ready access to all the equipment that may be required to access the airway is provided when the patient is in a specialized unit. It was the author's practice to have the required equipment at the bedside, at least for the first 48 hours. A flexible bronchoscope, a series of small uncuffed endotracheal tubes, usually a 6.0, 6.5, and 7.0, would be readily available. A small flexible bronchoscope can be placed through a 6.5 to 7.0 endo-tracheal tube to facilitate what might be a difficult intubation. A pediatric flexible bronchoscope can be readily passed through a number 6 endotracheal tube. If a "T" tube has been placed, the appropriate sized blue endotracheal tube connector should be taped to the bed rails. When the patient's airway is compromised, time should not be lost looking for the proper tubes and connectors. The reader is referred to the detailed chart outlined by Wooten and colleagues,[5] wherein the endotracheal blue connector size is matched to a variety of "T"-tube sizes. It is wise, however, to check that the blue adapter properly fits the T tube while the patient is still in the operating room.

Prophylactic Measures

There are several prophylactic measures to consider in order to prevent airway obstruction in the immediate postoperative period. There is no question that controversy exists as to the efficacy of several of the interventions discussed later. Many have simply been the product of experience in the larger centers. There are few properly conducted trials.

Humidified oxygen
Many of these patients will have hypoxia, as both a result of the procedure itself due to retained secretions and postoperative atelectasis and preexisting lung disease. With regards to the latter group, there will always be those patients who undergo tracheal resection secondary to postintubation tracheal stenosis and as a result of tracheostomy required for prolonged ventilator therapy. Several of these will have residual ventilation-perfusion mismatch and/or carbon dioxide retention. The latter group will be sensitive to any increase in the percentage of inhaled oxygen, and thus, the fraction of inhaled oxygen will require careful assessment. Close monitoring of oxygen saturation will be required, and in the hypercarbic group, one should aim for saturation

between 86% and 92%. This group will generally tolerate saturations less than 90%. Humidification is of course extremely important, and most particularly in those patients who require either a temporary tracheostomy or T tube.

Heliox and racemic epinephrine
Although both of these treatment modalities have been largely used in the management of croup or epiglottis, they have been observed to be beneficial when airway obstruction is secondary to edema of the anastomosis or the glottis. Helium is an inert, nontoxic, and low-density gas. Its low density decreases turbulence of air flow through a narrow channel. It can be delivered with oxygen as 70% to 80% helium and 20% to 30% oxygen. Beyond 30% oxygen, the laminar flow benefits of helium begin to decrease, and by 40% oxygen, most of the benefit is dissipated. Thus, if there is a significant ventilation-perfusion mismatch, helium may not be of benefit. Racemic epinephrine nebulization has been shown to decrease edema in cases of croup in children and epiglottis in adults. The usual dose in children according to UpToDate is 0.05 mL/kg per dose of a 2.25% solution diluted to 3 mL with saline. In adults, one uses 0.5 mL of a 2.25% solution diluted in 2.5 mL saline. The author has usually used racemic epinephrine and heliox together. Weber and colleagues[6] reported in a randomized trial in children with croup that both modalities were of equal benefit when used separately, but unfortunately, they did not have a group that received the 2 treatments concomitantly, to determine if the effects were additive.

Some tracheal surgeons use racemic routinely following subglottic resections or when a laryngeal drop has been used in order to prophylactically treat glottic or anastomotic swelling when such is not protected by a T tube.

Steroids and diuretics
Although some tracheal surgeons will use steroids routinely after subglottic resections,[4] such is not common practice given their defined effect on wound healing. The Harvard group,[3] like Toronto, avoids them as a routine measure but will add them if subglottic edema is persistent or symptomatic. Under such circumstances, a pulse of high dose (20–40 mg/d) over a short period of 5 to 7 days is best because such can be discontinued without tapering, and the long-term effects on wound healing should be avoided. It is notable that in their 2004 retrospective review of prognostic factors affecting anastomotic complications, Wright and colleagues[7] did not note any effect of steroids on anastomotic complications. No doubt

the steroid issue will continue to be better defined over time. In that regard, Shadmehr and colleagues[8] in a recent double-blind randomized trial noted a nonstatistical benefit of corticosteroids (15 mg/d) in the management of postintubation strictures. Patients receiving daily steroids had a longer interval between bronchoscopic dilatations, and there was a decreased incidence of required surgeries (28 of 50 in the steroid group and 40 of 50 in the nonsteroid group required surgery).

As with any surgery on the lungs or respiratory tract wherein respiratory difficulties postoperatively are not infrequent, the judicious use of diuretics is a valuable adjunct and can not only reduce anastomotic swelling but also decrease the accumulation of pulmonary interstitial water secondary to the anticipated alterations in pulmonary capillary permeability that follow.

Antiemetics

As with any general anesthetic and surgical procedure, nausea and vomiting in the immediate postoperative period are not uncommon. The prevention of regurgitation and vomiting is however especially important following tracheal surgery in an effort to prevent laryngeotracheal aspiration. The patient's ability to protect the airway is frequently compromised secondary to glottic dysfunction secondary to altered glottic movement, sensation, or vocal cord dysfunction. In addition, in major resections wherein a chin suture has been used to decrease anastomotic tension, the protective postural response to vomiting and or regurgitation is impaired.

Speech pathologist

Both speech and swallowing can be problematic in the early days following tracheal resection. The frequency of such difficulties is related to the length of the resection, the presence of a T tube (or tracheostomy tube), and the presence of vocal cord dysfunction. In the author's experience, such is especially the case when a laryngeal drop has been used or in cases of cricoid resection. If the upper arm of a T tube extends through the vocal cords, aspiration may be common during swallowing.

A speech pathologist is a valuable member of the team who can not only assist the patient in communication techniques but also make important recommendations to assist effective swallowing and prevent aspiration.

Bronchoscopy

As noted earlier, ready access to a variety of flexible bronchoscopes of various sizes, including pediatric scopes, is a prerequisite. The surgeon need be familiar with not only flexible scopes but also the use of various size rigid bronchoscopes. The indications for the use of a rigid scope in the immediate postoperative period are few, and if required, best done in the operating room, where control of the airway with anesthetic assistance is advisable. Nonetheless, the ability to use the rigid instrument in situations of airway obstruction not amenable to a flexible bronchoscope, without damaging the surgical site, is essential.

Although surveillance bronchoscopy will be required further into the postoperative period, there are several situations wherein the airway should be accessed:

- The presence of stridor is an absolute indication for bronchoscopic intervention. It is important to realize that stridor is rarely present until airway patency is more than 50% compromised. Although the appearance of stridor can occur for reasons other than a significant obstruction of the airway, an assessment of the cause is extremely important to ensure that any required intervention is undertaken before the situation becomes more extreme.
- Not only will the patient experience augmented tracheal and airway secretions, but also his or her ability to clear them are impaired especially if the glottis has been transgressed or the recurrent laryngeal nerve or nerves are damaged. Even when there is a T tube or small tracheostomy tube, suctioning may not be sufficient. Visualization and the use of saline lavage can greatly improve the situation. Repeated bronchoscopy is not uncommon in the first few days.
- Hypoxemia may be secondary to a variety of causes. On occasion, the ventilation/perfusion mismatch may be secondary to airway obstruction, which may be in the distal airway from accumulated secretions. It may also occur in the more proximal airway at the surgical site or even in a T tube despite the absence of stridor. An increasing fraction of inspired oxygen (Fio_2) should always lead to a visual examination of the airway unless there is obvious parenchymal disease to account for the hypoxemia.
- The presence of subcutaneous emphysema is an ominous sign usually indicative of anastomotic disruption. A thorough bronchoscopic examination will permit the surgeon to determine the required intervention, which will usually involve some form of anastomotic stenting. In severe cases of airway separation, especially if such occurs in the early post-

operative period, the flexible bronchoscope can be utilized to safely advance the endotracheal tube beyond the disruption.

- In the ventilated patient, any significant increase in airway pressure suggests that bronchoscopy is warranted to rule out obstruction amenable to bronchoscopic intervention. Although the author usually recommends bronchoscopy in any ventilated patient when airway pressures are increasing, it is even more important in the patient who has recently undergone any form of airway reconstruction. Maintaining low airway pressures is extremely important in order to prevent barotrauma to the anastomosis.

Bronchoscopy should be nontraumatic if undertaken with care. Before starting the procedure, the patient should be preoxygenated by increasing the Fio_2 for 5 minutes. In the awake patient without a T tube or tracheostomy, the transnasal route is best. Lidocaine spray 4% is liberally used in the nares and the back of the throat. A 1% or 2% lidocaine solution can then be injected through the scope once the vocal cords are visualized and again at intervals in the trachea and main stem bronchi. The transnasal route is essential in the patient, with a chin stitch given the degree of neck flexion.

In the presence of a T tube, bronchoscopy can be performed via the tube itself. Adequate lubrication is important to facilitate easy passage of the scope. Adequate lubrication can be achieved by initially injecting 2% lidocaine into the horizontal limb of the tube and applying liberal lubricant to the scope. It is possible to push the T tube into the airway if there is excessive pressure applied by the operator. To avoid this and permit the scope to pass easily, one can grasp the horizontal limb with a hemostat at the level of the skin incision to apply counterforce. Having a T tube in place not only makes airway access easier but also permits assisted ventilation during the procedure. A blue endotracheal tube connector of the appropriate size can be inserted into the horizontal limb opening and connected to an Ambu bag with the plastic diaphragm on the top of the connector to permit an airtight passage of the bronchoscope. A thorough examination of the entire airway is ensured simply by rotating the scope as it transcends the horizontal limb either cephalad or distally. One can assess the position of the upper limb relative to the vocal cords and assess vocal cord mobility. The size of the T tube determines the size of the bronchoscope.

As noted, bronchoscopy not only provides a visual assessment of the airway but also can also be used to alleviate obstruction. Following tracheal reconstruction, secretions are abundant, and often aspirated blood that migrated distally may continue to cause problems over the first few days following surgery. Saline lavage will usually be sufficient to clear the airway. However, if there is retained blood clot, simple lavage and aspiration may not be sufficient. Under those circumstances, a small-caliber Fogarty catheter can be passed down the suction channel, advanced beyond the clot, and then retracted once the balloon is inflated. Granulation tissue at the suture line has been noted in the past[4,7] to cause obstruction or the inspissation of secretions that may be troublesome. This problem is less frequent than in the past due largely to improvement in the type of suture material and surgical technique. Pearson always used fine wire sutures on the back wall of the anastomosis using a single square knot with the ends of the wire cut flush on the knot. Following that innovation, anastomotic granulation was exceedingly rare. However, if granulations are troublesome, they can be handled through judicious use of the flexible bronchoscope. Wooten and colleagues[5] report the use of a topical antibiotic steroid (ciprofloxacin and dexamethasone) to control granulations once identified either at the anastomosis or at the end of a T tube.

Ventilation

Although it is infrequently necessary, ventilatory support may at times be required. Tracheal strictures may be the result of a previous prolonged ventilation with an endotracheal tube or tracheostomy. Such patients often have some degree of underlying pulmonary disease that may predispose them to respiratory failure following tracheal reconstruction. Extensive laryngotracheal resections or those involving the tracheal carina may be prolonged and may also result in extensive soiling of the airway with residual secretions, which in addition to predisposing to airway obstruction may also lead to postoperative pneumonia. Particularly in the patient with impaired pulmonary reserve, moderate deterioration in ventilation-perfusion matching can lead to significant hypoxemia. The presence of a tracheal suture line complicates both intubation and the selection of the mode of ventilation.

Intubation

An awake intubation is preferred. Such is particularly important because often the indication for airway access is obstruction. Thus, it is important that spontaneous breathing be preserved. Deep sedation can be achieved without compromising respiratory effort. A benzodiazepine or propofol may be used. Propofol provides superb sedation and amnesia while maintaining patient cooperation and spontaneous respiration, usually in a dose of 2–2.5 mg/kg in an otherwise healthy adult (approximately 40 mg every 10 seconds until the onset of induction). It is the author's drug of choice when performing rigid bronchoscopy in the face of significant airway obstruction but is just as useful in facilitating intubation after tracheal reconstruction. Surgeons unfamiliar with its use are advised to have anesthesia involved, but the mechanics of the intubation is only for the surgeon to undertake when a fresh airway anastomosis is present.

When intubation is undertaken following airway resection, it should be performed under bronchoscopic guidance. Even when obstruction is not anticipated, visualization of the glottis and vocal cords may be difficult. Such is especially true following subglottic resections when there is considerable glottic edema for several days. In addition, it is extremely important for the surgeon to ensure that the tube is placed appropriately relative to the anastomosis or, if present, an indwelling T tube. If a chin stitch has been used, a laryngoscope is awkward and the cords difficult to view. For this reason and for ease of the procedure in the awake patient, the nasal route is best. A standard sized adult flexible bronchoscope can usually be inserted through a 6.5- or 7-mm endotracheal tube. If a smaller endotracheal tube is required, then a pediatric scope may be necessary. Following local anesthesia to the nares, pass the bronchoscope through the endotracheal tube first and then insert the scope into the nose. Ensure that the latex diaphragm is already in place on the endotracheal tube connector. Thus, once the tube is through the cords, the assistant can commence ventilation with an Ambu bag without an air leak while the surgeon carefully positions the tube relative to either a tracheal anastomosis or an indwelling T tube. Once the vocal cords are visualized, the scope facilitates the injection of further local anesthetic liberally on the glottis. If the patient has been well preoxygenated, there should be time to wait for the local anesthetic to affect the glottis, hence making passage of the scope easy. Once into the airway, advance the bronchoscope well into the airway before sliding the endotracheal tube through the glottis.

One of the common errors in such bronchoscopic intubation is when the surgeon advances the endotracheal tube and the bronchoscope together. The bronchoscope serves as a guide and a stent for the endotracheal tube, and passage of the latter is much easier once the former is well into the airway. The only situation when such is not advisable is when it has been determined that you do not wish the endotracheal tube to pass through the anastomosis.

When a T tube is in place, intubation may not be necessary. There are however circumstances wherein ventilation cannot be achieved with the T tube in place without intubation (see later discussion), and yet it is still desirable to leave the T tube in situ to protect the anastomosis. Such would be the case when the T tube is positioned across a subglottic anastomosis or when the T tube has been placed across a tracheal anastomosis that has undergone partial dehiscence. Once again, the bronchoscopic intubation provides the visualization required to properly place the lower end of the endotracheal tube. Depending on the relative size of the T tube and the endotracheal tube, it may be possible to pass the endotracheal tube into the upper limb of the T tube and obturate the airway without use of the endotracheal cuff. When anticipating such a maneuver, the endotracheal tube size should be assessed with a same-sized T tube as the one in the patient before intubation. If the T tube is high in the airway, securing the endotracheal tube may be difficult. A technique the author has found useful is as follows. Through the horizontal limb of the T tube, pass a small-caliber Fogarty catheter cephalad until it passes out the glottis and is visible in the mouth. Suture the end of the Fogarty catheter to the end of the endotracheal tube or tie it through the "eye" of the endotracheal tube. Use the bronchoscope as before to effect intubation by gently pulling on the Fogarty catheter. The traction on the Fogarty catheter actually facilitates the intubation to the point that the bronchoscope is used more to verify the endotracheal tube position than to actually effect the passage through the glottis. Once the endotracheal tube is properly placed either just above the T tube or into its upper limb, the Fogarty catheter is left in place while the silicone plug of the T tube is firmly inserted. The plug maintains the position of the endotracheal tube and provides the seal against further volume loss during ventilation.

Mode of ventilation

The selection of ventilation mode is particularly important when an airway anastomosis is present. The avoidance of high airway pressure is essential to reduce barotrauma. Likewise, endotracheal tube cuffs will need to remain uninflated, or if inflated, managed with some modicum of air leak to ensure that tracheal mucosal blood flow is not impaired and further airway damage is avoided, remembering that many of these patients acquired their tracheal pathologic condition following ventilation with cuffed tubes.

Ventilation without a T tube Most modern ventilators have a variety of available modes that facilitate ventilation with low peak airway pressures. An attempt should be made to support the patient with peak pressures less than 25 cm H_2O. Maintaining an air leak by either underinflating or simply not inflating the endotracheal tube cuff ensures that the tracheal mucosa is protected from the harmful effects of the cuff itself.

Ventilation in the face of a significant air leak can usually be adequately managed by either increasing the rate of ventilation or adopting a policy of permissive hypercapnia. The latter is an extremely useful technique. It is achieved by allowing the partial pressure of carbon dioxide (Pco_2) to increase gradually to provide time for metabolic compensation to occur. In practice, once the patient's ventilation is stabilized following intubation, the cuff is gradually deflated and the rate is increased. As the CO_2 increases gradually, metabolic compensation should allow the patient's pH to be safely maintained at no more than a moderate respiratory acidosis. Once intubated, the patient should be left with an air leak and ventilated with a high respiratory rate in order to permit a satisfactory minute ventilation with a low volume. Careful monitoring of arterial blood gases and peak airway pressures will allow the surgeon to gradually make adjustments in ventilatory parameters with the goal of permitting an ongoing air leak and low peak airway pressures while at the same time maintaining adequate oxygenation in the face of hypercapnia as long as the pH is greater than 7.2.

High-frequency jet ventilation (HFJV) is another viable option when air leaks are high and may permit normal Pco_2 when permissive hypercapnia is untenable or oxygenation cannot be adequately achieved with other means of low-pressure ventilation. Although such can readily be undertaken through a standard uncuffed endotracheal tube, the author has been concerned that sheer forces may be applied to the tracheal anastomosis, although this has not been properly documented. Thus, when using HFJV, it may be advisable to do through a catheter after positioning the tip of the catheter beyond the anastomosis. Effective ventilation can still be achieved.

Ventilation with a T tube The presence of a T tube complicates ventilation, because in most circumstances, it should not be removed in lieu of an endotracheal tube or a tracheostomy tube. Nonetheless, there are several techniques that permit the presence of the T tube while ventilation is in progress.

As noted above, it is possible to insert an endotracheal tube either just above the T tube or in some circumstances into the upper limb of the T tube. As the upper limb of the T tube will often be close to the glottis, dislodgement of the endotracheal tube is a concern. Securely anchoring the endotracheal tube can be achieved as mentioned above by the use of a Fogarty catheter. Under these circumstances, volume cycled/low-pressure ventilation can still be achieved. When ventilation is required with a T tube in place that is subglottic or through the cords, an alternative method would be the use of a laryngeal mask.

There are however other techniques one can use if intubation from above is difficult or undesirable. First, one can still use volume cycled/low-pressure ventilation with or without permissive hypercapnia. The upper limb can be occluded with a small-caliber Fogarty catheter passed cephalad as described earlier. The balloon is inflated in the upper limb of the T tube. A blue endotracheal tube connector of the correct size, which, as described earlier, should already be at the bedside, is inserted into the horizontal limb of the T tube and then connected to the ventilator tubing. The blue connector, if fitting snuggly, should prevent the distal migration of the Fogarty balloon, especially as air flow will actually tend to force it cephalad. If a large air leak subsequently ensues, then migration cephalad and out of the T tube has likely occurred. If airway pressures suddenly increase, then simply deflate the balloon and readjust the catheter's position. One other way to eliminate or reduce the air leak is to apply a tight-fitting continuous positive airway pressure (CPAP) mask to the patient's face and then ventilate via the T-tube horizontal limb, applying CPAP to the tight fitting mask.

HFJV or oscillation can also be used simply by advancing a small catheter down the distal limb of the T0 tube and into the trachea. As a T tube is usually beyond the anastomosis itself, sheer forces on the anastomosis are avoided.

The author has at one time or another used all these techniques and found that, although they all generally work well, one may find that in a particular patient a given technique is more effective. Success depends on a host of factors, including pulmonary compliance, airway resistance, the presence of preexisting hypercapnia, and the degree of ventilation/perfusion mismatch. As a result, failure to achieve adequate ventilatory support with one technique does not preclude trying some of the others. The important message is that ventilation can be safely undertaken while still protecting the tracheal suture line. Thus, when progressive respiratory failure is noted, prepare for all eventualities and do not delay ventilatory support when it is clearly required because of concerns that the surgical site might be damaged. Indeed, a respiratory arrest and hemodynamic collapse will produce far more tracheal damage, especially if establishing ventilation circuitry is traumatic because of the rush created by the emergency situation, particularly because several of the techniques noted earlier will be a novel experience.

SUMMARY

Most patients who undergo tracheal resections experience few complications. As Wright and colleagues[7] noted several years ago, the incidence of anastomotic complications has decreased over the years with improved suture technique and the development of superior suture materials. In addition, a more thorough appreciation of the methods for decreasing anastomotic tension has contributed to this improvement. At the same time, the ability to remove longer segments of airway and to extend resections into the larynx proper has managed to create novel situations that will require attention to postoperative management.

Prophylaxis is extremely important to enable the patient to avoid the need for assisted ventilation and to assure a long-term excellent result. However, when complications, either at the anastomotic site or from respiratory failure, ensue, the surgeon will need to be familiar with the techniques described in this article. In the author's opinion, the operating surgeon needs to be completely comfortable in the various bronchoscopic techniques described. In addition, the surgeon also needs to understand the importance of avoiding any intubation technique or ventilatory mode that might result in anastomotic trauma either directly or secondary to increases in airway pressure. Innovation is the key, and if the various techniques described above prove insufficient, keeping these principles in mind will enable other novel approaches to be developed.

REFERENCES

1. Grillo HC, Zannini P, Michelassi F. Complications of tracheal reconstruction. Incidence, treatment, and prevention. J Thorac Cardiovasc Surg 1986;91: 322–8.
2. Montgomery WW. Silicone tracheal T-tube. Ann Otol Rhinol Laryngol 1974;83:71–5.
3. Auchincloss HG, Wright CD. Complications after tracheal resection and re-construction: treatment and prevention. J Thorac Dis 2016;8(suppl 2): S160–7.
4. D'Andrilli A, Ciccone AM, Ventuta F, et al. Long term results of larnygo-tracheal resection for benign stenosis. Eur J Cardiothorac Surg 2008;7:227–30.
5. Wooten CT, Rutter MJ, Dickson JM, et al. Anesthetic management of patients with tracheal T-tubes. Paediatr Anaesth 2009;19(4):349–57.
6. Weber JE, Chudnofsky CR, Younger JG, et al. A randomized comparison of helium-oxygen mixture (Heliox) and racemic epinephrine for the treatment of moderate to severe croup. Pediatrics 2001; 107(6):E96.
7. Wright CD, Grillo HC, Wain JC. Anastomotic complications after tracheal resection: prognostic factors. J Thorac Cardiovasc Surg 2004;128:731–9.
8. Shadmehr MB, Abbasidezfouli A, Farzangan R, et al. The role of systemic steroids in post intubation tracheal stenosis: a randomized trial. Ann Thorac Surg 2017;103(1):246–53.

Prophylaxis and Treatment of Complications After Tracheal Resection

Paulo Francisco Guerreiro Cardoso, MD, MSc, PhD*,
Benoit Jacques Bibas, MD, Helio Minamoto, MD, PhD,
Paulo Manuel Pêgo-Fernandes, MD, PhD

KEYWORDS

• Tracheal diseases • Surgery • Complications • Prophylaxis • Treatment

KEY POINTS

- Tracheal resections are major surgical procedures that require a multidisciplinary approach involving thoracic surgery, anesthesiology, interventional airway endoscopy, otolaryngology, intensive care therapy, and speech pathology.
- Adequate patient selection and preparation may include interim procedures and correction of major comorbidities to achieve a successful outcome.
- Early and late postoperative complications may ensue and usually derive from local (ie, length of stenosis) and/or systemic (ie, diabetes) factors.
- Complications must be recognized and dealt with accordingly, based on its severity, and it may affect the long-term outcome.
- Cornerstones for prophylaxis of complications are meticulous patient selection, surgical planning and accurate technique, standardized postoperative care, and full patient awareness of the procedure.

INTRODUCTION

Tracheal stenosis is a complex surgical problem. It is frequently mistaken and interpreted as being a simple structural disease defined anatomically by its extension, diameter, and distance from the closest anatomic landmark, such as the vocal folds or the tracheal carina. In fact, tracheal stenosis is a heterogeneous disease in its cause, natural history, and clinical outcome.[1] It derives from various clinical entities, such as iatrogenic airway injuries (ie, postintubation, post-tracheostomy), autoimmune diseases (ie, Wegener granulomatosis, relapsing polychondritis, sarcoidosis, amyloidosis), congenital, primary and secondary neoplastic diseases, and idiopathic.

Postintubation tracheal stenosis still represents the most common indication for tracheal resection worldwide. Airway resection with primary reconstruction remains the definitive treatment modality for benign and malignant tracheal diseases.

The nature of airway surgery is challenging. It requires surgical expertise and skill in interventional endoscopic airway procedures. The advancements in tracheal surgery achieved after decades of research and solid clinical experience have ultimately led to an increase in the number of resections worldwide. Likewise, there has been an increase in the number of postresection complications ranging from 5% to 44%.[2–5] Identification of

Disclosure: The authors have nothing to disclose.
Division of Thoracic Surgery, Heart Institute Hospital das Clinicas da Faculdade de Medicina da Universidade de Sao Paulo (InCor-HCFMUSP), Rua Dr. Eneas de Carvalho Aguiar 44, bloco 2, 7° andar, Sao Paulo, Sao Paulo 05403-904, Brazil
* Corresponding author.
E-mail address: cardosop@gmail.com

Thorac Surg Clin 28 (2018) 227–241
https://doi.org/10.1016/j.thorsurg.2018.01.008

predictors for complications after tracheal resection, such as comorbidities, technical issues, and other factors, deserves consideration when a patient undergoes selection for a resection. There is a convergence between many of the predictors for complications in different centers.[3,4] The largest series ever published is a single-institution retrospective review of 901 patients who underwent tracheal resection at the Massachusetts General Hospital in Boston.[6] Complications occurred in 164 patients (18.2%) and half of the complications were anastomotic. At our institution, the complication rate was higher (44%) with 16% restenosis and 23% of nonanastomotic-related complications. The presence of comorbidities, previous resection, the extent of the resection, and laryngotracheal resections were related to a higher complication rate.[4] Higher anastomosis and redo tracheal resection are more prone to complications. Macchiarini and colleagues[7] described early complications in 41% of the patients submitted to a partial cricoidectomy with primary thyrotracheal anastomosis. Marulli and colleagues[8] reported 45.9% complications after laryngotracheal resections. The same authors reported a higher complication rate among idiopathic laryngotracheal stenosis (66.6%). An earlier large series of 75 redo tracheal resections reported a complication rate of 39% with a predominance in the group of patients submitted to previous laryngeal release maneuvers (63%).[9] The early detection of complications followed by a structured course of action in a timely fashion is critical for a successful outcome. Nowadays, the widespread use of computed tomography (CT) scan and bronchoscopy plays an important role in detecting complications and assessing its severity. Postresection complications and mortality vary across the series in different centers (**Table 1**).

IMPACT OF COMORBIDITIES

Clinical comorbidities are important risk factors on multivariate analysis in our cohort of complications after tracheal resections. Metabolic diseases and cardiovascular are the most frequently found in this population.

Diabetes

Diabetes is notorious for damaging the microcirculation and for its negative impact on wound healing. The nature of central airway resection and anastomosis includes a critical healing area in the presence of some degree of tension between the ends and a rather poor vascular supply. Such factors, when combined with a diseased microvascular bed secondary to diabetes, can triple the number of airway anastomotic complications,

Table 1
Postresection complications and mortality in different centers

Author, Date	Patients (N)	Complications (%)	Mortality (%)
Couraud,[10] 1994	217	4.6	3.2
Donahue et al,[9] 1997	75	39	2.6
Macchiarini et al,[7] 2001	45	41	2
Rea,[11] 2002	65	12.3	1.5
Wright et al,[6] 2004	901	18.2	1
Amoros,[12] 2006	54	9.2	1.8
D'Andrilli et al,[13] 2008	35	14.3	0
Marulli et al,[8] 2008	37	8.1	0
Cordos,[14] 2009	60	13.3	5
Bibas et al,[4] 2014	94	44.6	0

particularly anastomotic dehiscence after tracheal resection (odds ratio, 2.72; 95% confidence interval, 1.53–4.82; $P = .0004$).[3,6] In our cohort, the presence of diabetes was the most prominent comorbidity (45%).[4]

Obesity

Obesity is a risk factor in itself for prolonged mechanical ventilation. A meta-analysis comparing obese (body mass index ≥ 30 kg/m^2) with nonobese patients demonstrated that obesity in critically ill patients was not associated with excessive mortality but with prolonged duration of mechanical ventilation.[15] There are no prospective studies on the impact of obesity on the outcome of tracheal resection in tracheal stenosis and it varies across the series. There are, however, interesting studies on tracheostomy patients. A study on critically ill morbidly obese patients (body mass index ≥ 40 kg/m^2) submitted to tracheostomy showed an incidence of 25% complications compared with 14% in the nonmorbidly obese patients. On multivariate analysis, the morbid obesity was independently associated with a four-fold increased risk of tracheostomy-related complications.[15] Wright and colleagues[6] found that obesity (body mass index ≥ 30 kg/m^2) was not a risk factor for complications. In our cohort[4] the same criteria for obesity was related to a high risk of complications on the univariate analysis (odds ratio, 6.95; 95% confidence interval, 1.40–34.52; $P = .024$).

Cardiovascular

Coronary artery disease, arrhythmia, and stroke

It is estimated that approximately 12% of patients who undergo noncardiac surgery have or are at risk for coronary artery disease.[16] The combination of hypoxemia and tachycardia in patients with tracheal obstruction and coronary artery disease can interfere with the O$_2$ supply and demand. In this scenario, the rupture of a vulnerable coronary plaque can occur resulting in myocardial ischemia and infarction without an elevation of the ST segment. The mortality can be 15% to 25%.[17] Older patients must undergo screening for ischemic heart disease as part of their planning for tracheal resection. Protective measures must be taken to minimize the risk of an ischemic heart event in the perioperative period. However, patients with a previous history of cardiovascular events have a higher chance of developing a new one after a tracheal resection. Friedel and colleagues[18] described that 2 out of 110 (1.8%) tracheal resection patients who had a myocardial infarction in the past had another postoperative myocardial infarction and died. Two (1.8%) other patients developed intraoperative ventricular fibrillation and one died in the early postoperative period. One (0.9%) patient with a previous history of stroke and reanimation suffered a new stroke and died. Stroke can follow complex tracheal resections in elderly patients who had traction of the great vessels in the mediastinum during surgery (**Fig. 1**).

Pulmonary embolism

Postintubation tracheal stenosis is often found in patients who suffered a severe trauma and other conditions that require prolonged intubation and ventilatory assistance. Likewise, patients with major trauma have a high risk of thromboembolic events.[19] A study in a large trauma patient population showed that mechanical ventilation for more than 3 days was an independent factor for increasing the risk of thromboembolism up to 10-fold.[20] The correlation between venous thromboembolism and pulmonary embolism is frequent and must be kept in mind when patients develop tracheal stenosis because of its impact on the treatment strategy. This correlation is probably underdiagnosed and has been published as case reports.[21]

Gastroesophageal Reflux

Airway-related problems in patients with gastroesophageal reflux (GER) has a prominent inflammatory component associated with the presence of neutrophilic, neuroendocrine, inflammatory cells, and cytokines causing airway inflammation, and increased oxidative stress.[22] There are clinical studies in other airway diseases, such as pulmonary fibrosis, bronchiectasis, and asthma, showing a higher incidence of GER.[23–25] The association between laryngopharyngeal reflux and subglottic stenosis has been described particularly in patients with idiopathic tracheal stenosis.[26–29] There is a study suggesting that gastric juice can induce tracheal injury by means of tissue remodeling through the stimulation of the differentiation of fibroblasts into myofibroblasts.[30] Tawfik and colleagues[31] reported in a cohort of patients submitted to laryngotracheal resection that the presence of GER was associated with decannulation failure in those who required stenting. After a successful outcome with anti-GER disease therapy reported in a patient with idiopathic tracheal stenosis,[32]

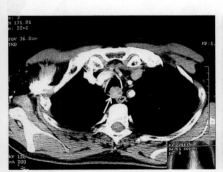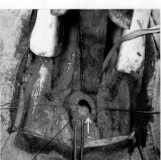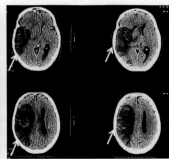

Fig. 1. A 73-year-old man submitted to transternal resection of squamous carcinoma of the trachea. (*Left*) CT scan showing the tumor (*arrow*). (*Center*) Transternal resection of the tumor (*arrow*). (*Right*) Extensive right hemisphere stroke after resection attributed to traction to the brachiocephalic artery (*arrows*).

we expanded the evaluation of GER to other patients with benign tracheal stenosis. Our preliminary data on esophageal manometry and 24-hour pH studies performed in patients with benign tracheal stenosis showed a high prevalence of abnormal acid reflux exposure (42%) with a predominance of supine reflux with a high upper esophageal acid exposure. This occurred with a low incidence of typical GER symptoms and in the presence of normal esophageal motility in most of the patients.[33] To date there are no studies on the prevalence of GER in patients with recurrences of the stenosis after tracheal resection. Such findings altogether suggest that GER may have an impact in the outcome of tracheal stenosis and deserve further investigation.

EARLY COMPLICATIONS
Bleeding

Severe bleeding after tracheal resection is a rare event. In our series of complications after tracheal resection, 2% of the patients had small hematomas in the neck.[4] However, large hematomas can cause severe discomfort and require intervention for evacuation for prevention of airway compression and edema (**Fig. 2**). At our center, the routine is to carry out a thorough hemostasis revision at the surgical site before wound closure. We do not routinely drain the incision after tracheal resection because there is no evidence that this causes impact on hematoma formation. Early reports showed a 1% rate of massive bleeding after tracheal resection, but most were caused by innominate artery hemorrhage.[34] Recent

publications have not reported severe bleeding episodes or reintervention because of bleeding.[13–35]

Dysphagia and Aspiration Pneumonia

Dysphagia and aspiration pneumonia are not frequent after tracheal and laryngotracheal surgery (2.6% and 4.2%).[2,4] Nevertheless, one must be aware of their occurrence particularly after high resections, such as subglottic resection, redo operations, laryngotracheal resections, and repair of a tracheoesophageal fistula (TEF) (**Fig. 3**).

The pathophysiology of postoperative swallowing dysfunction is complex, often multifactorial, and the onset of each cause is either concurrent or isolated. The predisposing factors are:

- Previous neck radiotherapy scarring or fibrosis derived from previous procedures
- Laryngeal edema causing coordination dysfunction
- Suprahyoid release impairing normal laryngeal excursion during swallowing
- Long segment tracheal resection preventing normal laryngeal elevation
- Recurrent laryngeal nerve palsy
- Advanced age
- Presence of a transglottic Montgomery T-tube
- High tracheal or laryngotracheal resections

The presence of a stent in the airway worsens the dysphagia symptoms. Lennon and colleagues[36] reviewed 38 patients submitted to laryngotracheal

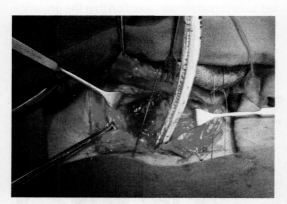

Fig. 2. A 38-year-old man who submitted to a subglottic resection developed respiratory discomfort on the first postoperative day. Rexploration of the cervical incision showed a hematoma adjacent to the right thyroid lobe causing laryngeal displacement and airway compression. Note the "guardian stitches" in place.

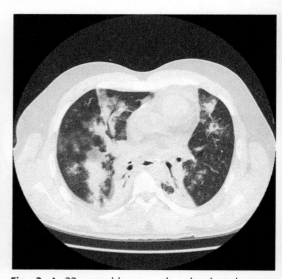

Fig. 3. A 32-year-old man who developed severe aspiration pneumonia on the third postoperative day after a redo tracheal resection.

resection and found a mean duration of postoperative dysphagia of 8 days in patients who had a stent in place as opposed to 4.8 days in patients who had not. In regards to the need for a feeding tube, the duration of dysphagia symptoms was 3.7 days in patients who had a stent but did not require a feeding tube in the long term, as opposed to 50.8 days in those who required a feeding tube. Whenever dysphagia and aspiration are detected in the early postoperative period, immediate interruption of the oral intake and placement of a feeding tube is required. Most the patients recover within the next 2 to 3 weeks and rarely require placement of a long-term gastrostomy tube to maintain nutrition. In many patients with no previous symptoms, dysphagia can occur during the first aspiration episode in the early postoperative period.

Although aspiration pneumonia can ensue regardless of the age of the patient, older patients and patients with previous dysphagia are more prone to aspirate as a result of the impairment of airway protective reflexes (ie, swallowing and cough reflexes).[37] In such instances a thorough evaluation of the swallowing function preoperatively is warranted. Postoperatively, elderly patients who underwent suprahyoid laryngeal release procedure are also at risk for aspiration. A modified barium swallow study can reveal the extent and severity of the swallowing dysfunction.

The swallowing mechanism tends to improve with time and exercise, but enteral feeding may be required. Sihag and Wright[3] described in their large series that 2.6% of patients submitted to airway resection developed a swallowing dysfunction with aspiration. At our center, dysphagia is also not frequent (4.2%), and aspiration pneumonia has been a rare event after tracheal and laryngotracheal resection. For high resections, such as subglottic, laryngotracheal, or redo resections, the patients receive tutoring by the speech pathologist postoperatively during their first meals. If any signs of aspiration are detected, oral diet is suspended temporarily and a modified barium swallow is performed. If aspiration is unequivocal in the contrast study, a nasogastric-feeding catheter is put in and the patient is assessed and followed by a speech pathologist thereafter. Those patients who remain unable to resume oral diet after 3 to 4 weeks undergo a percutaneous endoscopic gastrostomy. The percutaneous endoscopic gastrostomy procedure has shown to be safe and effective, although the complication rate is not negligible in large retrospective and prospective series (13% and 27%, respectively). The most frequent complications after percutaneous endoscopic gastrostomy are diarrhea, leakage, and peristomal infection.[38,39]

Laryngeal Dysfunction

Obstructive edema
Obstructive edema is more common after laryngotracheal resection and reconstruction as opposed to tracheal resection. Obstructive airway symptoms often derive from laryngeal edema with obstructive swelling and voice change. The symptoms are dyspnea, stridor, and swallowing dysfunction.

Recurrent laryngeal nerve injury
This is a rare complication that accounts for less than 2% in the reported series that include laryngotracheal resections where the nerve is adjacent to the field of dissection.[3] The strategy to prevent laryngeal nerve injury is to dissect in the peritracheal plane immediately adjacent to the airway to avoid violating the tracheoesophageal groove. We routinely make no effort to identify the path of the recurrent nerve during a tracheal resection.

Hoarseness
This requires investigation with direct laryngoscopy. Even if there is immobility of one of the vocal cords, the potential for recovery is not known. However, if there is any objective evidence of aspiration in a patient with a suspected recurrent nerve injury, an assessment and follow-up by the speech pathologist is warranted to improve swallowing and phonation. Mild hoarseness requires low-dose steroids, nebulized epinephrine, voice rest, and head elevation. Like dysphagia, the improvement of hoarseness occurs with time and help of the speech pathologist. If airway obstruction is a concern, intubation with a small, uncuffed endotracheal tube is recommended. If edema fails to resolve after a few days of intubation and medical therapy, one must consider a tracheostomy. Likewise, the detection of bilateral vocal cord palsy postoperatively secondary to recurrent laryngeal nerve injury is an indication for tracheostomy because of risk of glottis obstruction.

Paraplegia and Tetraplegia

Paraplegia and tetraplegia are rare disastrous complications after tracheal resection mentioned in the literature mostly in case reports. The mechanisms described involve neck hyperflexion, mechanical compression by osteophytes, spinal cord ischemia, and systemic hypotension. In 1981, Borrelly and colleagues[40] reported a case of paraplegia in a female patient who underwent tracheal resection through sternotomy for resection of an adenoid cystic carcinoma of the trachea. The "guardian stitch" (chin-to-chest) was used.

The patient experienced a transient loss of movement and sensibility in the lower limbs in the early postoperative period that resolved spontaneously 2 days later. The same patient underwent another tracheal resection 1 year later and had paralysis of the left leg postoperatively. This time it lasted 5 days and the leg movements returned but a hypoesthesia remained for 30 months. A CT scan revealed compression of the spinal cord by a large osteophyte of the cervical column. In another report, a patient underwent transternal resection for adenoid cystic carcinoma and experienced arterial hypotension in the first postoperative day.[41] The guardian stitch was used and in the second day after surgery, a paralysis of both legs was noticed after extubation. The removal of the guardian stitch reversed the paralysis. There is also a dramatic report by Dominguez and coworkers in 1996[42] on a tracheal resection and neck hyperflexion using the guardian stitch where the patient was placed in a sitting position postoperatively and developed tetraplegia a few hours later that did not reverse. The suggested mechanism was spinal cord ischemia involving the sitting position,[43] which was refuted by Grillo.[44] A case of spinal cord ischemia after cricotracheal resection was reported in a patient who also had the guardian stitch but with the head kept in neutral position.[45] The patient developed irreversible tetraplegia on the sixth postoperative day. It apparently resulted from spinal cord edema and infarction, although the exact cause of injury remained unclear. The authors suggested that despite the rareness of such events, it should be included in the informed consent because of its severity and long-term implications.

Anastomosis Dehiscence

Anastomotic separation is a feared and serious complication of tracheal resection. Separation of the suture line to some degree was detected in less than 1% of patients in the Massachusetts General Hospital experience.[3,6] Our group also reported anastomotic dehiscence in 1% of patients in a smaller series.[4] It occurs within the first days or weeks after surgery, and excessive tension in the anastomosis is frequently the main cause for dehiscence. The resulting defect is often found in the anterior aspect of the anastomosis where most of the tension is located.[2] Clinically, patients present with dyspnea and stridor of variable severity and subcutaneous emphysema and wound infection. The detection of any sign of anastomotic separation or dehiscence prompts for an immediate evaluation that includes a neck and chest CT scan followed by a flexible

bronchoscopy in the operating room. The priorities are to check the viability of the anastomosis and to secure the airway. A small dehiscence in a patient that breathes comfortably and with no signs of major complications in the neck incision, such as bleeding or abscess formation, requires no surgical revision. Antibiotic therapy is then started and drainage of the neck incision is performed to control local contamination.[2] Anastomotic separations larger than 5 mm frequently require surgical management, especially if the patient is symptomatic. In this scenario concomitant laryngeal edema is often present (**Fig. 4**).

Securing the airway in a patient with cervical inflammation and laryngeal edema after a recent laryngotracheal resection is a challenging endeavor. Our choice is to perform a bronchoscopy-guided intubation in the operating room under general anesthesia as follows. The procedure starts with face-mask ventilation, followed by an evaluation of the airway performed either by flexible bronchoscopy or by rigid tracheoscopy using a suspension laryngoscope and a 5 mm/30° rigid telescope.[46] Flexible bronchoscopy is difficult in this setting because of laryngeal edema and abundant secretions. We prefer to use the rigid scope because it allows a thorough examination of the larynx and enables a safer and straightforward intubation through the anastomosis under direct vision. A number 5.5F catheter or 6.0F catheter cuffed endotracheal tube placed over the rigid optical telescope is pushed down the suspension laryngoscope. Once advanced into the larynx and into the proximal trachea, the endotracheal tube is slid over the telescope and its end placed beyond the anastomosis.

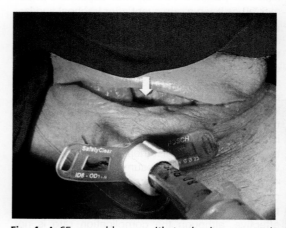

Fig. 4. A 65-year-old man with tracheal anastomosis dehiscence (*arrow*) after a tracheal resection and reconstruction. Dehiscence was treated successfully with a tracheostomy and a complete open drainage of the cervicotomy. (*Courtesy of* Messias Froes Jr, MD, Heart Institute-InCor HCFMUSP, Sao Paulo, Brazil.)

The criticism of this approach is the need for a neck extension that poses additional strain to the anastomosis that is already open and will require a tracheostomy anyway. Any attempts of intubation with the patient awake or breathing spontaneously can be disastrous and shall be avoided at all costs. With the patient intubated, the neck incision is explored and a tracheostomy constructed either at the dehisced anastomosis or just below it. A neck CT scan and a flexible bronchoscopy programmed for the next 3 to 4 weeks after the tracheostomy clarifies the local healing status. If healing is considered adequate, the tracheostomy cannula is substituted by a silicone T-tube because of its ability to restore airway patency and phonation while a proper healing of the underlying anastomosis takes place.[47,48] All efforts must converge to avoid losing the recently reconstructed airway. If severe laryngeal edema is still present, a supraglottic silicone T-tube may be required for a short period (6 months), and changed for another T-tube placed below the vocal folds to improve speech. Long-term silicone stenting after surgery in this scenario yields to good a surgical outcome, and removal of the T-tube should be attempted after another 6 to 12 months.[3,6,48]

Wound Infection

Cervical wound infection affects 10% of the patients submitted to tracheal resection.[4] Skin redness, purulent discharge through the incision, and cervical pain are suggestive signs and symptoms of a wound infection.[2] Concomitant cough, increased sputum production, or stridor associated with a wound infection should raise the suspicion of anastomotic separation. A chest and neck CT scan should be performed to check for any anastomotic problems, such as extra luminal air or undrained fluid collection (**Fig. 5**).[2] Initial treatment consists of broad-spectrum intravenous antibiotics followed by drainage of the cervical

incision if there is fluctuation or purulent discharge through the incision. If an anastomotic dehiscence is suspected, an urgent bronchoscopy done in the operating room is followed by the therapeutic measures described previously in the section on anastomosis dehiscence. When diagnosis and treatment are started in a timely fashion, a better outcome and complete resolution are expected in the long term. It is advisable to evaluate the patency and diameter of the anastomosis with a CT scan up to 1 year after successful treatment (**Fig. 6**).

Subcutaneous and Mediastinal Emphysema

The onset of subcutaneous emphysema is abnormal after a tracheal or a laryngotracheal resection. It is by definition a surrogate for an anastomotic complication. The detection of subcutaneous emphysema within the first 2 days after a tracheal resection can represent an early leak in the anastomosis, and often results from a tense suture line. Moreover, progressive subcutaneous emphysema occurring 3 to 5 days after surgery raises the suspicion of an anastomosis dehiscence, and requires an urgent evaluation of the airway. A small asymptomatic mediastinal emphysema might be present in chest CT scan after a low tracheal resection, and requires simple observation if the patient is breathing normally. Nonetheless, the presence of extraluminal air with any signs of respiratory discomfort or distress must prompt for an urgent endoscopic and radiologic evaluation.

Tracheoinnominate Artery Fistula

This is a devastating complication with low incidence (0.7%) but a high mortality which can be in excess of 75%.[49,50] Grillo and colleagues[34] described five cases of postoperative tracheoinnominate fistula (TIF) in a series of 521 tracheal

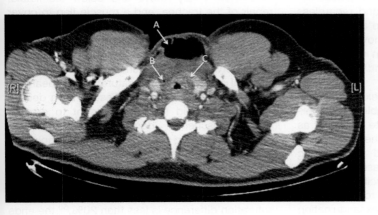

Fig. 5. A 40-year-old woman 5 days after a tracheal resection and reconstruction. Axial neck CT scan shows signs of a contained anastomosis leak represented by (A) cervical and (B) peritracheal air collection; anastomotic edema (C). Clinical inspection showed signs of wound infection.

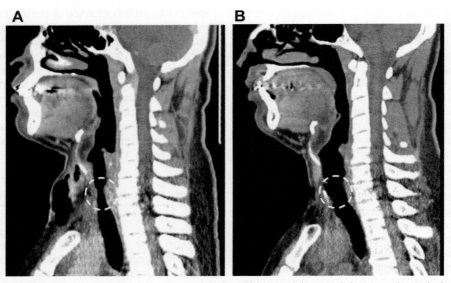

Fig. 6. Same patient as in **Fig. 5.** Patient was treated with antibiotics and cervical drainage through the neck incision. Sagittal CT scan of the neck and chest before (*A*), and 1 year after treatment (*B*) showing complete resolution and a preserved diameter of the anastomosis (*dashed circles*).

resections for postintubation stenosis with three deaths (two had anastomotic separation, one managed with repair of the artery, and the other by division of the innominate artery). Postresection TIF can derive from an infection in the surgical site, particularly when lower resections are performed through the neck in addition to a tracheostomy below the anastomosis. The mechanism involves the erosion of the artery and a communication with the tracheal wall. The outcome depends mostly on a combination of factors that include (1) early diagnosis, (2) immediate control of the hemorrhage, (3) maintain airway patency, (4) expedite surgical management, and (5) the type of repair performed.[51] The diagnosis is based on a clinical suspicion after an initial bleeding episode (sentinel bleeding) either by hemoptysis or via the tracheostomy cannula. Such bleeding episode occurs in 35% to 50% of the patients and, regardless of its magnitude, it must be valued and warrants investigation.[52,53] Bronchoscopy shows a pulsatile bare area in the tracheal wall. On CT scan the innominate artery is adjacent to and/or displaced by the trachea (**Fig. 7**).

Because the risk of bleeding and exsanguination is always imminent and unpredictable, it is imperative to proceed with the immediate treatment as soon as the diagnosis is established. However, the presence of an active and catastrophic bleeding requires bedside local measures directed to control the bleeding and resuscitation before taking the patient to the operating room because of the high risk of asphyxia and exsanguination

during transport. In patients with a tracheostomy or an endotracheal tube, overinflation of the balloon cuff is the first measure resulting in successful temporary control of the bleeding in 85% of the cases.[53] Stoma hemorrhage is controlled by digital compression of the innominate artery against the manubrium through the tracheostomy.[54] Airway control must be achieved in the operating room by bronchoscopy-guided intubation or hyperinflation of the tracheostomy cuff. In patients with a tracheostomy, a better local control of the bleeding is achieved using a wired silastic tracheostomy cannula with an adjustable wing. This facilitates the position of the overinflated cuff over the bleeding site to provide temporary hemostasis.[51] The surgical management of TIF includes a median sternotomy with the division of the innominate artery above and below the fistula, repair of the trachea, and a muscle flap to cover the oversewn vessels (**Fig. 8**).[55]

To minimize cerebral ischemia, the monitoring of cerebral blood flow uses the blood pressure difference between the bilateral radial arteries and regional cerebral oxygen saturation by means of near-infrared spectroscopy. Testing for a decline in cerebral blood flow is important to prevent cerebral ischemic damage. Furukawa and colleagues[51] used a 3-minute test clamping of the innominate artery to perform such test. On division of the innominate artery proximal and distal to the fistula, if the systolic pressure difference is within 30 mm Hg and the regional cerebral oxygen saturation difference is less than 20%,[56] the ends

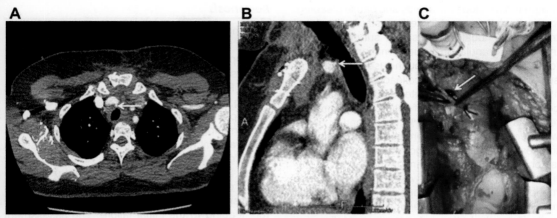

Fig. 7. A 27-year-old man with sentinel bleeding through the tracheostomy 28 days after tracheal resection. (*A*) Axial contrast chest CT scan. (*B*) Sagittal reconstruction showing innominate artery adjacent to the anterior tracheal wall with a small indentation (aneurism) suggesting a tracheoinnominate fistula (*arrows*). (*C*) Surgery: sternotomy with ligation of the innominate artery proximal and distal to the fistula; opening of the tracheal wall in the fistulous tract (*arrow*). (*Courtesy of* Celso M.N. Faria, MD and Isaac F.S. Rodrigues, MD, Faculdade de Medicina de Sao Jose do Rio Preto-FAMERP, Sao Paulo, Brazil.)

of the divided artery are oversewn. If the systolic radial pressure and cerebral blood flow shows a higher difference in the values, an innominate-to-innominate or innominate-to-right common carotid artery bypass is performed. One must be aware that in the presence of an infected operative site, either a primary repair of the innominate artery or an arterial bypass is to be avoided because both are at risk of graft infection and rebleeding.[52] Endovascular stenting of the innominate artery has emerged as a nonsurgical method for controlling the bleeding by covering the fistula site. After the initial report in 2001 by Deguchi and colleagues,[57] endovascular stenting has been

reported scarcely in the literature for the treatment of TIF. The current stent technology enables a less invasive approach but the risk of infection and TIF recurrence remain. The suggestion of stenting as a temporary measure before definitive surgical treatment[58] is discretionary in TIF and must be viewed with caution particularly in patients after tracheal resection.

LATE COMPLICATIONS AND MANAGEMENT
Granulomas

Granulation tissue formation at the level of the anastomosis is a local inflammatory process that can

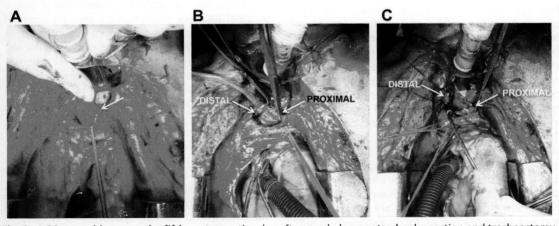

Fig. 8. A 36-year-old man on the fifth postoperative day after a redo laryngotracheal resection and tracheostomy. Patient had developed an infection in the surgical site and presented a massive in-hospital bleeding requiring resuscitation. (*A*) Finger compression of the bleeding site adjacent to the innominate artery (*arrow*). (*B*) Control of the bleeding site with proximal and distal clamps under extracorporeal circulation caused by rupture of the artery during dissection. (*C*) Proximal and distal stumps of the innominate artery divided and oversewn.

progress to occlude the airway and cause bleeding. In the past it was attributed mostly to the local trauma and local response to suture material. Indeed, the granulation tissue formation in the anastomosis reduced after the routine use of absorbable suture material. Grillo and colleagues[34] reported in 1995 that 1.6% of resected patients had this complication after the use of absorbable suture material, as opposed to 23.6% in the earlier series when polyester sutures were used. At our unit the tracheal-tracheal or laryngotracheal anastomosis is done using two polyglactin full-thickness stay sutures in both sides of the airway, and polydioxanone monofilament suture for separated or continuous running sutures of the posterior and anterior airway walls. Recently, better understanding of inflammation has shed light into other mechanisms potentially involved. Patients using stents after surgery are more prone to develop granulation tissue, possibly because of local irritation and colonization. Nouraei and colleagues[59] investigated the role of local colonization by microorganisms in patients using airway prosthesis and found a strong association between the occurrence of airway granulation and the presence of *Staphylococcus aureus* and *Pseudomonas aeruginosa*.

Tracheoesophageal Fistula

Tracheal resection is required during repair of a TEF in 41% to 60% of instances.[60] The recurrence of TEF may occur when tracheal resection is performed as part of the repair of a TEF.[60] The early recurrence of TEF after repair is a life-threatening complication.[61-63] In our series of patients with benign TEF, 55% needed a concomitant tracheal resection, 5% had a TEF recurrence, and 15% had recurrence of the tracheal stenosis.[64] Muniappan and colleagues[60] reported a similar recurrence rate (11%). Despite the scarcity of publications on predictors for TEF recurrence, previous attempted repairs, prior esophagectomy, and laryngectomy seem to be associated with poorer outcomes. The management of early TEF recurrence is complex because of local infection in addition to salivary aspiration and pneumonia. Treatment strategy depends on local factors, such as the extent of the TEF; infection; presence of a tracheal dehiscence; and the general clinical condition of the patient, which is often poor. A tracheostomy is frequently necessary in this scenario. Secondary TEF repairs are a challenging surgical undertaking even for an experienced surgeon. In our series, three patients had a prior TEF repair.[64] Only one had an uneventful recovery. The other two still have indwelling tracheal stents but are able to eat and breathe normally.

Restenosis

Restenosis occurs in less than 1% of patients submitted to resection and reconstruction.[3] However, the reported incidence may be underestimated because of the high rate of unreported restenosis.[65] Residual stenosis is a possibility in this setting, particularly if the resection was either incomplete or carried out in the presence of active inflammation of the tracheal margins. The patients with tracheal restenosis usually develop dyspnea and stridor within 2 to 4 weeks after the primary repair. Treatment of tracheal recurrent stenosis in such cases involves meticulous preoperative assessment of and a complete scrutiny of the factors leading to the initial failure. The assessment starts with a chart review of the first procedure. This can provide important information regarding the extent of previous resection, the surgical technique used, and the analysis of the potential factors that might have contributed to failure. Ideally, the second intervention should be deferred until the planning, complete clinical evaluation, and stabilization of comorbidities are taken care of. Meanwhile, the restenosis can be temporarily stented with placement of a T-tube or a straight Dumon silicone stent depending on the existence of a tracheostomy. A CT scan with multiplanar reconstruction is essential to assess any extraluminal component of the stenosis and its position in relation to the innominate artery and the other mediastinal structures. Laryngoscopy and bronchoscopy are performed as a separate procedure before reintervention. It helps guiding the decision to proceed or not with the reintervention. The key observations at laryngoscopy/tracheoscopy are (1) the length of stenosis, (2) the length of proximal and distal normal trachea, (3) presence of active tracheal mucosal inflammation, and (4) signs of vocal cord dysfunction. If active inflammation is evident at the resection margins of the restenosis, surgery is delayed for 6 months to allow inflammation and infection to subside. In the Massachusetts General Hospital series the average time interval between the initial operation to the redo resection was 8 months.[9] Our own series had 21% of anastomotic complications, in which 16% were restenosis treated endoscopically with dilatation and stenting (8.5% needed a T-tube and/or tracheostomy). All had achieved a successful outcome.[4] The T-tube insertion is the preferred method to optimize the airway because it minimizes inflammation, preserves speech, and is easy to manage.[65] Some patients with tracheal restenosis actually do well with the T-tube in the long-term. In a series of 140 patients who underwent T-tube placement, Gaissert and colleagues[66] described long-term use in 112 patients exceeding 1 year in 49 patients and 5 years in 12 patients.[66] In selected patients with inoperable benign tracheal stenosis, tracheal stenting could be used as a curative therapeutic approach. We reported a successful decannulation in 27.5% at 5 years (mean follow-up time of 34 months).[48] Redo resection comes into play when dilation fails to ensure airway patency. In restenosis, if there is an adequate segment of residual trachea for reconstruction, the success rate can reach 92% despite the increased risk of anastomotic complications and the need for 6 months to 1 year for complete resolution of postoperative healing.[9] Surgical technique is a determining factor for a successful reconstruction. The dissection kept close to the trachea is fundamental to preserve the lateral tracheal blood supply, the integrity of the recurrent laryngeal nerves, and the esophagus. The circumferential exposure of the trachea is necessary only at the level of the stenotic segment. In the redo operative field, the presence of scar tissue and limited amount of trachea available for reconstruction makes the surgeon's margin for error slim. This part of the dissection is done unhurriedly to avoid excessive anastomotic tension. As the surgical margins in benign restenosis are concerned, an abnormal margin of trachea may be accepted if the cartilage has a stable luminal diameter with a nonobstructive airflow. Our preference is to perform the anastomosis using interrupted 4-0 absorbable sutures (polyglactin or polydioxanone). If tension at the anastomosis is excessive, release maneuvers are performed liberally. About 25% of patients undergoing redo resection require release maneuvers, compared with 6% in primary resection.[9] Besides the neck flexion maneuver, the Montgomery suprahyoid release[67] is the most commonly used to reduce anastomosis tension because it is easy to do and provides a downward displacement of larynx and cervical trachea by up to 2 cm. The maneuver often results in temporary postoperative dysphagia. The hilar release by division of the inferior pulmonary ligament and pericardium adjacent to the inferior pulmonary vein can also be used. After redo resection, the patient needs monitoring in the intensive care unit for 24 to 48 hours. Postoperative flexible bronchoscopy is performed within 7 to 14 days of the operation to evaluate the anastomosis. The complication rate after redo resection is greater if compared with primary tracheal resection (39%).[9]

Predictors of Postoperative Complications

Defining the predictors of postoperative complications in tracheal resection is a way to discern which patients are at risk. There is some consensus in the literature regarding long-segment resections (>4 cm), obesity, and diabetes as high-risk factors for anastomosis failure.[4,6] Nevertheless, the odds ratio can vary depending on the target population, and the center and the surgical team's experience. Multivariate analysis is a helpful tool for determining the risk factors. Sihag and Wright[3] described that age less than 17 years, preoperative tracheostomy, long-segment resection, the need for an intraoperative release maneuver, laryngotracheal resection, and redo resections are significant risk factors. Diabetes increased the risk of anastomotic complications. The need for laryngotracheal resections is also associated with increased risk of complications. A recent series from Mexico with 155 patients[5] found that the presence of laryngeal stenosis was the only significant predictor for complications. The analysis of the predictors for complications in our series of 94 patients[4] showed that the most prominent risk factor for complications was the previous history of tracheal resection. The presence of comorbidities was also prominent and was justified by the high prevalence of diabetes (45%). Long-segment resection was also an ominous risk factor. This presence of peritracheal fibrosis from the previous resection reduces the tracheal mobility and increases anastomosis tension. **Table 2** summarizes the predictors of complications derived from multivariate analysis.

PROPHYLAXIS

The prevention of complications after tracheal resection starts with a correct indication for resection and a thorough preoperative evaluation and meticulous surgical technique. Expert anesthetic and postoperative care in centers where a trained multidisciplinary staff perform airway surgery routinely are the key issues for a successful airway surgery program.

Preoperative Preparation

Systemic steroids have a negative impact on wound healing of the tracheal anastomosis and should be weaned off before resection. Obesity also correlates with an increase in postoperative complications. Secretions or significant tracheobronchitis detected in preoperative bronchoscopy demands treatment with a course of antibiotics before surgery. Complete airway assessment must include the function of the vocal cords. Glottis dysfunction should be addressed before subglottic or tracheal surgery.

Technique

The basic technical principles of tracheal surgery must be strictly observed to prevent postoperative

Table 2
Predictors of complications derived from multivariate analysis

Author, Date Risk Factor	Multivariate Analysis		
	OR	95% CI	P Value
Sihag and Wright,[3] 2015			
Diabetes	2.7	1.53–4.82	.0004
Bibas et al,[4] 2014			
Previous tracheal resection	49.9	2.40–1.03	.012
Resection >4 cm	5.1	1.93–13.77	.001
Comorbidities	7.0	1.51–32.84	.013
Berrios-Mejía et al,[5] 2016			
Laryngotracheal resection	2.9	1.27–6.65	.011
Resection >4 cm	2.2	0.88–5.61	.090
Wright et al,[6] 2004			
Previous tracheal resection	3.0	1.69–5.43	.002
Diabetes	3.3	1.76–6.26	.002
Resection >4 cm	2.0	1.21–3.35	.007
Laryngotracheal resection	1.8	1.07–3.01	.03
Tracheostomy before resection	1.7	1.03–3.14	.04
Age <17 y	2.2	1.09–4.68	.03

Abbreviations: CI, confidence interval; OR, odds ratio.

complications. This includes (1) the preservation of the blood supply in the tracheal ends, (2) avoiding tension in the anastomosis using release maneuvers, and (3) good anastomotic technique and adequate absorbable suture material. The prophylaxis of early postoperative complications is also focused on slow diet advancement to prevent aspiration, aggressive clearance of secretions, voice rest for laryngotracheal resections, judicious use of the guardian chin stitch, and surveillance bronchoscopy. Laryngeal reconstruction can generate some degree of glottic edema and laryngeal dysfunction. Both can impact in the normal swallowing mechanism and pose a greater risk of postoperative aspiration. Patients with obstructive upper airway swelling, stridor, and airway compromise may need a temporary tracheostomy.

Airway Surgery Team

A multidisciplinary team is required to manage these complex patients. The team approach plays a major role in preventing and detecting complications and it does impact on the patient's outcome. At our division at the University of São Paulo, patients are seen and treated at the airway center. This is a concept that congregates a multidisciplinary team approach consisting of thoracic surgery, respiratory endoscopy, and pulmonology working alongside with the speech pathologists and otolaryngologists. This allows better and integrated care for patients with tracheal diseases, which is important in high-volume centers.

Redo Resections

Strict selection is the first step toward prevention of complications in a redo resection. Besides being a challenging surgical procedure, the redo resection remains the most important predictor for anastomotic complications after airway resection. The chance for complications after a redo resection is between 3 and 49 times higher than in the primary resection.[4,6] In fact, many patients are not actual candidates for the procedure because of insufficient residual tracheal length. Ideally, a redo operation should not be attempted before 6 months from the first procedure to allow peritracheal inflammation to resolve. Meanwhile, airway patency is maintained by stenting using silicone stents. However, the presence of a tracheostomy or a T-tube before a redo resection increases the chance of postoperative complications as a result of (1) colonization of the airways with pathogens, (2) placement of a tracheal stoma nearby the site of stenosis resulting in a second stenosis, and (3) scarring of the neck reducing the mobility of the trachea.[6]

Other Underlying Tracheal Diseases

Central airway stenosis is found in 10% to 16% of patients with Wegener granulomatosis, and in only 2% of cases it represents the primary manifestation of the disease.[68,69] Patients with Wegener granulomatosis are poor candidates for resection because of the unpredictable and relapsing course of their disease. Resection in patients with Wegener granulomatosis is scarcely reported in the literature and is reserved for patients with fixed lesions and long periods of disease quiescence.[70,71] Other autoimmune conditions, such as relapsing polycondritis, share a similar clinical course with multiple migrating stenoses and are likewise best managed by immunosuppression and repeat dilatation rather than resection.

Tracheal Stenosis and Concurrent Tracheoesophageal Fistula

These patients are at the highest risk for complications because they often have a long segment of involved trachea, chronic inflammation around the stenosis site, dense tracheal adhesions to the surrounding tissues, and a nutritional imbalance.[64] Prophylaxis includes improvement in nutrition and treatment of pulmonary infection and physiotherapy before scheduling surgical correction of the TEF.

Resectable Tracheal Tumors

If tracheal resection is feasible, the anticipated extent of the resection must be carefully planned along with reconstruction strategy that includes the approach and the need for release maneuvers. It is advisable to avoid radiation therapy preoperatively whenever possible because of the resulting dense fibrosis and damage to the local vascular supply.

REFERENCES

1. Gelbard A, Donovan DT, Ongkasuwan J, et al. Disease homogeneity and treatment heterogeneity in idiopathic subglottic stenosis. Laryngoscope 2016; 126(6):1390–6.
2. Auchincloss HG, Wright CD. Complications after tracheal resection and reconstruction: prevention and treatment. J Thorac Dis 2016;8(Suppl 2): S160–7.
3. Sihag S, Wright CD. Prevention and management of complications following tracheal resection. Thorac Surg Clin 2015;25(4):499–508.
4. Bibas BJ, Terra RM, Oliveira Junior AL, et al. Predictors for postoperative complications after tracheal resection. Ann Thorac Surg 2014;98(1):277–82.
5. Berrios-Mejía J, Morales-Gómez J, Guzmán-de Alba E, et al. Resección traqueal y laringotraqueal en estenosis traqueal: factores predictores de recurrencia posoperatoria. Neumol Cir Torax 2016;75(4): 275–80.
6. Wright CD, Grillo HC, Wain JC, et al. Anastomotic complications after tracheal resection: prognostic factors and management. J Thorac Cardiovasc Surg 2004;128(5):731–9.
7. Macchiarini P, Verhoye JP, Chapelier A, et al. Partial cricoidectomy with primary thyrotracheal anastomosis for postintubation subglottic stenosis. J Thorac Cardiovasc Surg 2001;121(1):68–76.
8. Marulli G, Rizzardi G, Bortolotti L, et al. Single-staged laryngotracheal resection and reconstruction for benign strictures in adults. Interact Cardiovasc Thorac Surg 2008;7(2):227–30 [discussion: 30].
9. Donahue DM, Grillo HC, Wain JC, et al. Reoperative tracheal resection and reconstruction for unsuccessful repair of postintubation stenosis. J Thorac Cardiovasc Surg 1997;114(6):934–8 [discussion: 8–9].
10. Couraud L, Jougon J, Velly JF, et al. Iatrogenic stenoses of the respiratory tract. Evolution of therapeutic indications. Based on 217 surgical cases. Ann Chir 1994;48(3):277–83.
11. Rea F, Callegaro D, Loy M, et al. Benign tracheal and laryngotracheal stenosis: surgical treatment and results. Eur J Cardiothorac Surg 2002;22(3): 352–6.
12. Amoros JM, Ramos R, Villalonga R, et al. Tracheal and cricotracheal resection for laryngotracheal stenosis: experience in 54 consecutive cases. Eur J Cardiothorac Surg 2006;29(1):35–9.
13. D'Andrilli A, Ciccone AM, Venuta F, et al. Long-term results of laryngotracheal resection for benign stenosis. Eur J Cardiothorac Surg 2008;33(3):440–3.
14. Cordos I, Bolca C, Paleru C, et al. Sixty tracheal resections–single center experience. Interact Cardiovasc Thorac Surg 2009;8(1):62–5 [discussion: 5].
15. Akinnusi ME, Pineda LA, El Solh AA. Effect of obesity on intensive care morbidity and mortality: a meta-analysis. Crit Care Med 2008;36(1):151–8.
16. Mangano DT, Wong MG, London MJ, et al. Perioperative myocardial ischemia in patients undergoing noncardiac surgery–II: incidence and severity during the 1st week after surgery. The Study of Perioperative Ischemia (SPI) Research Group. J Am Coll Cardiol 1991;17(4):851–7.
17. Devereaux PJ, Goldman L, Yusuf S, et al. Surveillance and prevention of major perioperative ischemic cardiac events in patients undergoing noncardiac surgery: a review. CMAJ 2005;173(7): 779–88.
18. Friedel G, Kyriss T, Leitenberger A, et al. Long-term results after 110 tracheal resections. Ger Med Sci 2003;1:Doc10.
19. Geerts WH, Code KI, Jay RM, et al. A prospective study of venous thromboembolism after major trauma. N Engl J Med 1994;331(24):1601–6.
20. Knudson MM, Ikossi DG, Khaw L, et al. Thromboembolism after trauma: an analysis of 1602 episodes from the American College of Surgeons National Trauma Data Bank. Ann Surg 2004;240(3):490–6 [discussion: 6–8].
21. Tzouvelekis A, Kouliatsis G, Oikonomou A, et al. Post-intubation pulmonary embolism and tracheal stenosis: a case report and review of the literature. Respir Med 2008;102(8):1208–12.
22. Carpagnano GE, Resta O, Ventura MT, et al. Airway inflammation in subjects with gastro-oesophageal reflux and gastro-oesophageal reflux-related asthma. J Intern Med 2006;259(3):323–31.
23. Bandeira CD, Rubin AS, Cardoso PF, et al. Prevalence of gastroesophageal reflux disease in patients with idiopathic pulmonary fibrosis. J Bras Pneumol 2009;35(12):1182–9.
24. Machado Mda M, Cardoso PF, Ribeiro IO, et al. Esophageal manometry and 24-h esophageal pH-metry in a large sample of patients with respiratory symptoms. J Bras Pneumol 2008;34(12):1040–8.

25. Fortunato GA, Machado MM, Andrade CF, et al. Prevalence of gastroesophageal reflux in lung transplant candidates with advanced lung disease. J Bras Pneumol 2008;34(10):772–8.

26. Blumin JH, Johnston N. Evidence of extraesophageal reflux in idiopathic subglottic stenosis. Laryngoscope 2011;121(6):1266–73.

27. Maronian NC, Azadeh H, Waugh P, et al. Association of laryngopharyngeal reflux disease and subglottic stenosis. Ann Otol Rhinol Laryngol 2001;110(7 Pt 1):606–12.

28. Jindal JR, Milbrath MM, Shaker R, et al. Gastroesophageal reflux disease as a likely cause of "idiopathic" subglottic stenosis. Ann Otol Rhinol Laryngol 1994;103(3):186–91.

29. Little FB, Koufman JA, Kohut RI, et al. Effect of gastric acid on the pathogenesis of subglottic stenosis. Ann Otol Rhinol Laryngol 1985;94(5 Pt 1):516–9.

30. Jarmuz T, Roser S, Rivera H, et al. Transforming growth factor-beta1, myofibroblasts, and tissue remodeling in the pathogenesis of tracheal injury: potential role of gastroesophageal reflux. Ann Otol Rhinol Laryngol 2004;113(6):488–97.

31. Tawfik KO, Houlton JJ, Compton W, et al. Laryngotracheal reconstruction: a ten-year review of risk factors for decannulation failure. Laryngoscope 2015; 125(3):674–9.

32. Terra RM, de Medeiros IL, Minamoto H, et al. Idiopathic tracheal stenosis: successful outcome with antigastroesophageal reflux disease therapy. Ann Thorac Surg 2008;85(4):1438–9.

33. Cardoso PFG, Trindade JM, Nasi A, et al, editors. Prevalence of gastro-esophageal acid reflux in benign upper airway stenosis. 19 WCBIP/WCBE. Florence (Italy): World Association of Bronchology and Interventional Pulmonology; 2016.

34. Grillo HC, Donahue DM, Mathisen DJ, et al. Postintubation tracheal stenosis. Treatment and results. J Thorac Cardiovasc Surg 1995;109(3):486–92 [discussion: 92–3].

35. D'Andrilli A, Maurizi G, Andreetti C, et al. Long-term results of laryngotracheal resection for benign stenosis from a series of 109 consecutive patients. Eur J Cardiothorac Surg 2016;50(1):105–9.

36. Lennon CJ, Gelbard A, Bartow C, et al. Dysphagia following airway reconstruction in adults. JAMA Otolaryngol Head Neck Surg 2016;142(1):20–4.

37. Ebihara S, Ebihara T, Kohzuki M. Effect of aging on cough and swallowing reflexes: implications for preventing aspiration pneumonia. Lung 2012;190(1): 29–33.

38. Blomberg J, Lagergren J, Martin L, et al. Complications after percutaneous endoscopic gastrostomy in a prospective study. Scand J Gastroenterol 2012; 47(6):737–42.

39. Lee C, Im JP, Kim JW, et al. Risk factors for complications and mortality of percutaneous endoscopic gastrostomy: a multicenter, retrospective study. Surg Endosc 2013;27(10):3806–15.

40. Borrelly J, Simon C, Bertrand P. Cases of regressive paraplegia after repeated resection of the trachea - one case. Ann Chir 1981;35(8):618–9.

41. Pitz CC, Duurkens VA, Goossens DJ, et al. Tetraplegia after a tracheal resection procedure. Chest 1994;106(4):1264–5.

42. Dominguez J, Rivas JJ, Lobato RD, et al. Irreversible tetraplegia after tracheal resection. Ann Thorac Surg 1996;62(1):278–80.

43. Dominguez J, Rivas JJ, Lobato RD, et al. Tetraplegia after tracheal resection. Ann Thorac Surg 1997; 64(2):583.

44. Grillo H. Invited commentary. Ann Thorac Surg 1996; 62:278–80.

45. Windfuhr JP, Dulks A. Spinal cord infarction following cricotracheal resection. Int J Pediatr Otorhinolaryngol 2010;74(9):1085–8.

46. Santos AO Jr, Minamoto H, Cardoso PF, et al. Suspension laryngoscopy for the thoracic surgeon: when and how to use it. J Bras Pneumol 2011; 37(2):238–41.

47. Bibas BJ, Bibas RA. A new technique for T-tube insertion in tracheal stenosis located above the tracheal stoma. Ann Thorac Surg 2005;80(6): 2387–9.

48. Terra RM, Bibas BJ, Minamoto H, et al. Decannulation in tracheal stenosis deemed inoperable is possible after long-term airway stenting. Ann Thorac Surg 2013;95(2):440–4.

49. Shepard PM, Phillips JM, Tefera G, et al. Tracheoinnominate fistula: successful management with endovascular stenting. Ear Nose Throat J 2011;90(7): 310–2.

50. Grillo HC, Mathisen DJ. Cervical exenteration. Ann Thorac Surg 1990;49(3):401–8 [discussion: 8–9].

51. Furukawa K, Kamohara K, Itoh M, et al. Operative technique for tracheo-innominate artery fistula repair. J Vasc Surg 2014;59(4):1163–7.

52. Gelman JJ, Aro M, Weiss SM. Tracheo-innominate artery fistula. J Am Coll Surg 1994;179(5): 626–34.

53. Jones JW, Reynolds M, Hewitt RL, et al. Tracheoinnominate artery erosion: successful surgical management of a devastating complication. Ann Surg 1976;184(2):194–204.

54. Utley JR, Singer MM, Roe BB, et al. Definitive management of innominate artery hemorrhage complicating tracheostomy. JAMA 1972;220(4):577–9.

55. Ridley RW, Zwischenberger JB. Tracheoinnominate fistula: surgical management of an iatrogenic disaster. J Laryngol Otol 2006;120(8):676–80.

56. Samra SK, Dy EA, Welch K, et al. Evaluation of a cerebral oximeter as a monitor of cerebral ischemia during carotid endarterectomy. Anesthesiology 2000;93(4):964–70.

57. Deguchi J, Furuya T, Tanaka N, et al. Successful management of tracheo-innominate artery fistula with endovascular stent graft repair. J Vasc Surg 2001;33(6):1280–2.

58. Palchik E, Bakken AM, Saad N, et al. Endovascular treatment of tracheoinnominate artery fistula: a case report. Vasc Endovascular Surg 2007;41(3):258–61.

59. Nouraei SA, Petrou MA, Randhawa PS, et al. Bacterial colonization of airway stents: a promoter of granulation tissue formation following laryngotracheal reconstruction. Arch Otolaryngol Head Neck Surg 2006;132(10):1086–90.

60. Muniappan A, Wain JC, Wright CD, et al. Surgical treatment of nonmalignant tracheoesophageal fistula: a thirty-five year experience. Ann Thorac Surg 2013;95(4):1141–6.

61. Macchiarini P, Verhoye JP, Chapelier A, et al. Evaluation and outcome of different surgical techniques for postintubation tracheoesophageal fistulas. J Thorac Cardiovasc Surg 2000;119(2):268–76.

62. Semlacher RA, Bharadwaj BB, Nixon JA. Management of a post-traumatic tracheo-esophageal fistula following failed primary repair. J Cardiovasc Surg (Torino) 1994;35(1):83–6.

63. Mathisen DJ, Grillo HC, Wain JC, et al. Management of acquired nonmalignant tracheoesophageal fistula. Ann Thorac Surg 1991;52(4):759–65.

64. Bibas BJ, Guerreiro Cardoso PF, Minamoto H, et al. Surgical Management of Benign acquired tracheoesophageal fistulas: a ten-year experience. Ann Thorac Surg 2016;102(4):1081–7.

65. Madariaga ML, Gaissert HA. Reresection for recurrent stenosis after primary tracheal repair. J Thorac Dis 2016;8(Suppl 2):S153–9.

66. Gaissert HA, Grillo HC, Mathisen DJ, et al. Temporary and permanent restoration of airway continuity with the tracheal T-tube. J Thorac Cardiovasc Surg 1994;107(2):600–6.

67. Montgomery WW. Suprahyoid release for tracheal anastomosis. Arch Otolaryngol 1974;99(4):255–60.

68. Gluth MB, Shinners PA, Kasperbauer JL. Subglottic stenosis associated with Wegener's granulomatosis. Laryngoscope 2003;113(8):1304–7.

69. Rasmussen N. Management of the ear, nose, and throat manifestations of Wegener granulomatosis: an otorhinolaryngologist's perspective. Curr Opin Rheumatol 2001;13(1):3–11.

70. Utzig MJ, Warzelhan J, Wertzel H, et al. Role of thoracic surgery and interventional bronchoscopy in Wegener's granulomatosis. Ann Thorac Surg 2002;74(6):1948–52.

71. Solans-Laque R, Bosch-Gil J, Canela M, et al. Clinical features and therapeutic management of subglottic stenosis in patients with Wegener's granulomatosis. Lupus 2008;17(9):832–6.

Nonoperative Endoscopic Management of Benign Tracheobronchial Disorders

Cameron D. Wright, MD

KEYWORDS

- Bronchoscopy • Airway stenting • Tracheal dilation

KEY POINTS

- Advanced bronchoscopy is a fundamental skill required by thoracic surgeons.
- Dilation of the airway is now most simply accomplished by balloon dilation.
- Stenting of the airway for benign lesions requires skill with a variety of techniques and stents.
- A variety of ablation therapies are available for advanced management of airway lesions.

Endoscopy of the airway is a fundamental skill required of thoracic surgeons who manage airway abnormality. The modern videobronchoscope has certainly made airway evaluation easier and allows all in the procedure room or operating room to be engaged in the procedure. Bronchoscopes come in several different sizes (diameters), including neonatal (3.1 mm), pediatric (4.2 mm), regular adult (4.8 mm), and therapeutic (6.2 mm). Therapeutic bronchoscopes with a larger therapeutic channel allow passage of larger biopsy forceps, balloon dilators, and laser and cryotherapy devices. Rigid bronchoscopy was almost a lost art but has been resurrected and is now a mainstay again for endoluminal therapy for the airway.[1,2] Rigid bronchoscopy allows ventilation, the use of large suction catheters for aspiration, removal of foreign bodies, passage of larger therapeutic devices into the airway, and use of the tip of the bronchoscope to debulk obstructing tumor quickly. Rigid bronchoscopes of varying sizes can also be used for serial dilation of tracheal stenoses. Rigid bronchoscopy requires close collaboration with the anesthesiologist and a thoughtful strategy for ventilation, either standard ventilation or jet ventilation. The introduction of a rigid bronchoscope into the airway is often a challenging procedure for novices. Simulators are available as well as videos to help teach this almost-lost art. Of course, general anesthesia is required for rigid bronchoscopy. Proper positioning is important with extension of the head and neck, and sometimes a shoulder roll is helpful to further extend the head. Protection of the teeth with a tooth guard is required. Suctioning of the airway before insertion of the bronchoscope is helpful, of course. The anesthesiologist should make sure the patient is well ventilated and oxygenated before attempting insertion to allow the surgeon a leisurely amount of time to access the airway. Some surgeons use a laryngoscope first to expose the supraglottic area, allowing easy passage of the rigid bronchoscope with a limited field of view into the airway. Others, the author included, prefer to introduce the rigid bronchoscope and use it as a fulcrum to elevate the back of the tongue, expose the supraglottic area, and then introduce the bronchoscope into the airway. This procedure is usually accomplished most easily from the midline of the mouth and is, of course, facilitated if the patient is edentulous. Alternatively, if the

Disclosure: The author has nothing to disclose.
Division of Thoracic Surgery, Massachusetts General Hospital, Harvard Medical School, Founders 7, 55 Fruit Street, Boston, MA 02114, USA
E-mail address: cdwright@mgh.harvard.edu

thoracic.theclinics.com

patient has somewhat protruding teeth, the surgeon can insert the bronchoscope from the lateral aspect of the mouth, which allows an easier plane of insertion into the airway.

AIRWAY STENOSIS

There are many causes of benign airway stenosis, and most of them are iatrogenic (**Box 1**). Extrinsic benign stenoses are usually treated by removal of the offending agent causing pressure on the airway. Intrinsic benign stenoses are usually treated by dilation, at least as an initial step in their management. Dilation can be done with gradually increasing sizes of rigid bronchoscopes, with plastic bougies of gradually increasing sizes, or by balloon dilation (**Fig. 1**). Balloon dilation has the advantage of being able to be performed with the therapeutic flexible bronchoscope and is the most common method of dilation now. The balloon dilators come in assorted sizes for accurate dilation diameters. One disadvantage of balloon dilation is there is no "feel" of the stenosis, so it is possible to overdilate and disrupt the airway if one is not careful. Postintubation tracheal stenosis is the commonest benign stenosis treated by bronchoscopic techniques. If patients are treated acutely, it is important to know as much about the airway as possible before therapeutic intervention. Sometimes a simple posterior-anterior and lateral chest radiograph will clearly show the area of stenosis and its length and the status of the distal trachea beyond the stenosis. More commonly, a computed tomographic (CT) scan is performed that will allow a much more precise estimation of

the location, length, and degree of stenosis. Typically a CT will underrepresent the degree of stenosis. The surgeon must make plans to control the airway if the patient is in any distress and must be ready to quickly dilate the airway to allow satisfactory ventilation. Tracheostomy beyond the lesion is rarely necessary because endoscopic techniques usually will rapidly reestablish an airway. Obviously, blind tracheostomy without knowing the status of the distal airway or where it is normal is to be avoided because opening the trachea in an area of stenosis is fraught with trouble and often leads to disaster. Especially close communication with the anesthesiologist is necessary when taking an acutely dyspneic patient with postintubation stenosis to the operating room for urgent airway dilatation. Dilations for circumferential postintubation tracheal stenosis typically are a temporizing measure only and will only last for several weeks (**Fig. 2**). For shorter stenoses with some preservation of native epithelium, it is often worthwhile to attempt a few dilatations to see if the stenosis will settle down into a comfortably dilated state and allow the patient to avoid a tracheal resection. However, if several dilatations fail to correct the problem and the patient has a short operable stenosis, referral should be made for tracheal resection. Posttracheostomy stomal stenoses typically do not respond to dilatation well but also happily are rarely severely symptomatic (**Fig. 3**). The pathophysiology of the formation of stenosis is, of course, different from a cuff stenosis, which is circumferential. Stomal stenoses occur because of necrosis and collapse of the anterior wall of the trachea, leading to an A-shaped stenosis. Typically, the lateral and posterior walls are relatively unaffected and have normal mucosa. Stomal stenosis are usually stable stenoses as opposed to circumferential cough stenoses, which often have abnormal epithelium or granulation tissue. Stomal stenoses do not dilate well because the membranous wall is typically quite flexible and stretches as a dilator is passed.

LASER THERAPY

Several lasers are useful for benign tracheobronchial disorders.[3] These lasers include the Nd:YAG, KTP, and thulium lasers. All 3 of these provide a good combination of hemostatic as well as cutting/vaporization effect. Lasers are quite helpful in clearing granulation tissue. Lasers are also helpful in conjunction with mechanical removal or to core out airway tumors. They can vaporize smaller tumors or treat the residual base of a tumor after mechanical removal. They are also useful to control bleeding at the base of a tumor. Laser safety

---

Box 1
Causes of benign central airway obstruction

Intrinsic

Postintubation tracheal stenosis

Posttracheostomy stomal stenosis

Anastomotic stricture

Granulation tissue

Tuberculosis, histoplasmosis, sarcoidosis

Amyloid

Papillomatosis

Tracheopathia osteoplastica

Relapsing polychondritis

Extrinsic

Lymphadenopathy: sarcoidosis, tuberculosis, histoplasmosis

Goiter

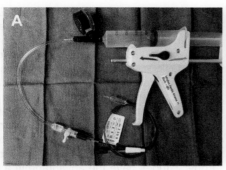
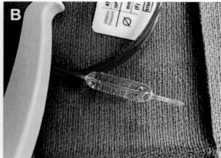

Fig. 1. (*A*) Balloon dilating system with gun and pressure gauge along with balloon. (*B*) Close-up view of balloon dilator.

procedures, of course, must be followed (**Box 2**). It is important in general to undertreat the base of a lesion because the laser heat penetrates several millimeters deeper than what is observed with the eye. The membranous wall should be treated with respect because it is so thin and the esophagus resides just below. Last, one must be cognizant of "past pointing" with the laser beam because the airway beyond the treated lesion can be injured.

CRYOTHERAPY

Spray cryotherapy is a relatively new modality useful in treating some airway disorders, including granulations, stenoses, foreign body removal, and tumors.[4,5] Liquid nitrogen at −196°F is delivered via a special flexible cryocatheter that can be passed via the working channel of a therapeutic bronchoscope. As the liquid changes to gas, it expands exponentially. When the gas is released at the tip of the bronchoscope, the intense cold causes a rapid freeze of surrounding exposed

airway and causes cell death and tissue necrosis. If spray cryotherapy is used, the necrosis is superficial, and underlying epithelial cells can repopulate the airway and lead to a more stable epithelium. Because of the exponential expansion of gas when the liquid nitrogen is converted to gas, adequate egress for the large volume of gas must be provided to prevent airway injury of a pneumothorax. An open rigid bronchoscope is probably best, although a laryngeal mask airway or an endotracheal tube with the cuff down and the circuit removed from the opening has been used. In addition, tight distal airway stenoses (ie, in the bronchus intermedius) should not be treated because the entrained gas distal to the stenosis has no room to expand and can lead to a pneumothorax.

ARGON PLASMA COAGULATION

Argon plasma coagulation uses argon gas and an electrical generator to create a stream of ionized gas that creates a superficial zone of coagulative

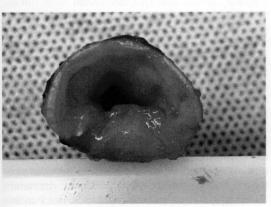

Fig. 2. Typical postintubation circumferential cuff stenosis.

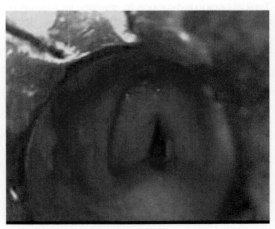

Fig. 3. Typical posttracheostomy stomal A-shaped stenosis.

necrosis that provides excellent hemostasis but very limited penetration.[6] Thus, it can be useful for small areas of granulation but is of limited use for debulking tumors.

ELECTROCAUTERY

Electrocautery is a contact energy modality that generates thermal energy from the flow of electrons from an electrical generator.[7] A variety of delivery devices can be used for ablation (a simple probe), cutting (scissors), and resection (snare). As with laser use, caution needs to be exercised to avoid airway fires with the use of low Fio_2 ventilation.

STENTING

Airway stenting is used most often with malignant airway obstructions but also has valuable uses in benign cases as well. Typically, an airway stenosis is first dilated (and/or lasered), and then a stent is inserted to maintain longer-term airway patency. Typical benign indications for stenting include unresectable postintubation tracheal stenosis, long-segment inflammatory stenosis (ie, sarcoidosis, tuberculosis), and post–lung transplant stenoses.

Walters and Wood[1] listed the ideal characteristics of an airway stent, as follows: (1) easily deployed and adjusted but does not migrate, (2) resists compressive forces yet does not erode or breach the native airway wall, (3) conforms to the airway without kinking or bending, (4) elicits minimal foreign body reaction and prevents tissue ingrowth or granulation, and (5) allows mucociliary clearance to decrease mucous impaction. As might be expected, there is currently no perfect stent.

The main types of stents are silicone and expandable.[8–10] Silicone stents come in 2 varieties, the tracheal T tube, which is inserted through a tracheostomy stoma, which holds it in place, and simple self-retaining stents, which typically have some sort of anchoring design to prevent migration (knobs or lips). Silicone stents are relatively inexpensive, are fairly easy to adjust and remove, and usually elicit minimal granulation tissue reaction. They come in many lengths and diameters. Disadvantages include an unfavorable inner-to-outer diameter ratio leading to relative airway narrowing; they can be compressed by a more rigid airway, and they can be challenging to deploy, requiring general anesthesia and rigid bronchoscopy. T tubes have the advantage (if a tracheostomy stoma is already in place) of being easy to change and can occasionally act as a healing stent, which allows the stenotic airway to remodel and stabilize around the silicone T tube, allowing its eventual removal. T tubes tend to be very airway friendly, and the underlying tracheal mucosa is usually not traumatized. However, they do require daily care with saline cleansing, and the anchoring capped T portion of the tube is unsightly. Self-retaining silicone stents have the advantage that no external portion is visible in the neck, and they rarely require changing once they are properly seated and located. They do often incite granulation tissue underneath the stent, which can be a problem if one wants to remove the stent. Silicone stents do not seat well in malacic airways and thus tend to migrate. Of course, silicone stents can be ignited by lasers, so caution must be used if a laser is used in conjunction with a silicone stent when granulations must be treated.

Self-expandable metal stents (SEMS) have a more favorable inner-to-outer diameter ratio and thus a larger resulting airway than silicone stents. They are relatively easy to place and can be delivered with the therapeutic flexible bronchoscope under local or general anesthesia, with or without fluoroscopy. Once deployed, SEMS rarely migrate. SEMS are typically made with nitinol, which further expands with warming to body temperature and can exhibit significant radial force. SEMS can be covered or uncovered. Uncovered stents allow tissue ingrowth but typically incite severe granulation tissue ingrowth and resulting airway obstruction. They are almost impossible to remove once in place for a while and are now rarely placed. Indeed, the US Food and Drug Administration issued a "Black Box" warning that bare metal airway stents should be avoided in the management of benign airway stenosis[11] (**Fig. 4**). Modern SEMS are covered with polyurethane and come in many different diameters and lengths. A variation on SEMS is the Polyflex (Boston Scientific, Marlborough, MA, USA) stent, which is just self-expanding and is made of

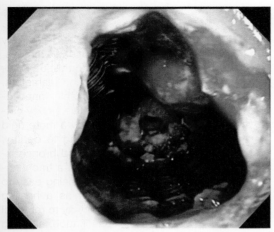

Fig. 4. Bronchoscopic view of an uncovered SEMS placed for postintubation tracheal stenosis with obstructing granulation tissue at the top and bottom of the stent as well as within the stent.

polyester covered with polyurethane. The stents are also easy to place and perhaps are more easily removed than SEMS.

REFERENCES

1. Walters DM, Wood DE. Operative endoscopy of the airway. J Thorac Dis 2016;8S:130–9.
2. Hsia D, Musani AI. Interventional pulmonology. Med Clin North Am 2011;95:1095–114.
3. Ramser ER, Beamis JF. Laser bronchoscopy. Clin Chest Med 1995;16:415–26.
4. Moore RF, Lile DJ, Abbas AE. Current status of spray cryotherapy for airway disease. J Thorac Dis 2017; 9S:122–9.
5. DiBardino DM, Lanfranco AR, Haas AR. Bronchoscopic cryotherapy. Clinical applications of the cryoprobe, cryospray and cryoadhesion. Ann Am Thorac Soc 2016;13:1405–15.
6. Morice RC, Ece T, Ece F, et al. Endobronchial electron beam plasma coagulation for the treatment of hemoptysis and neoplastic airway obstruction. Chest 2001;119:781–7.
7. Boxem T, Muller M, Venmans B, et al. Nd:YAG versus bronchoscopic electrocautery for palliation of symptomatic airway obstruction: a cost-effectiveness study. Chest 1999;116:1108–12.
8. Semaan R, Yarmus L. Rigid bronchoscopy and silicone stents in the management of central airway obstruction. J Thorac Dis 2015;7S:352–62.
9. Vavares MA. Tracheal T tubes for long-term management of the unreconstructable trachea in adults. Otolaryngol Head Neck Surg 2017;157:164–6.
10. Ayub A, Al-Ayoubi AM, Bhora FY. Stents for airway strictures: selection and results. J Thorac Dis 2017; 9S:116–21.
11. Lund ME, Force S. Airway stenting for patients with benign airway disease and the Food and Drug Administration advisory: a call for restraint. Chest 2007;132:1107–8.

Printed and bound by CPI Group (UK) Ltd, Croydon, CR0 4YY

08/05/2025

01864711-0006

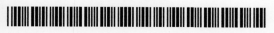